13-6'09

MASTERS RUNNING

MASTERS RUNNING

A GUIDE TO RUNNING AND STAYING FIT AFTER 40

HAL HIGDON,
AUTHOR OF
*MARATHON: THE
ULTIMATE TRAINING
GUIDE*

RODALE

NOTICE

Printed in the United States of America
Rodale Inc. makes every effort to use acid-free ∞, recycled paper ♻.

Book design by Drew Frantzen

Library of Congress Cataloging-in-Publication Data

Higdon, Hal.
    Masters running : a guide to running and staying fit after 40 / Hal Higdon.
       p.   cm.
    Includes index.
    ISBN-13 978–1–59486–021–8 paperback
    ISBN-10 1–59486–021–1 paperback
    1. Running for older people.   2. Physical fitness for older people.   I. Title.
GV1061.18.A35H55   2005
613.7'172'0846—dc22   2004027381

Distributed to the trade by Holtzbrinck Publishers

2   4   6   8   10   9   7   5   3   1   paperback

RUNNER'S WORLD ®

For the latest running news
and training tips, please visit us at
www.runnersworld.com

RODALE
LIVE YOUR WHOLE LIFE™

We inspire and enable people to improve their lives and the world around them
For more of our products visit **rodalestore.com** or call 800-848-4735

In memory of Paul Derr, Mike O'Connor, Cy DeCoster, Wally Hass, Ted Haydon, Frank McBride, and Fred Wilt, the coaches who made me a master runner.

CONTENTS

INTRODUCTION

MOTIVATION

We Define Our Own Goals and Levels of Success

In 1977, I traveled to Gothenburg, Sweden, to compete in the World Masters Championships, a track-and-field meet for older athletes. I ran well, winning the 3000-meter steeplechase and setting a world record for my age group: M45. I also placed third in the marathon and fourth in cross-country. But the hero of the championships was Duncan MacLean of Scotland, who won the 100 meters in what was then the oldest age group: M80.

MacLean's time of 21.27 was not what grabbed everybody's attention; it was his age. The Scot actually was 91 years old! Although even older participants would appear at future World Masters Championships (a 100-year-old runner competed in Australia in 2001), MacLean was the oldest at the time and also was ahead of his time. What impressed me about MacLean, who once had worked as an understudy for the famous singer Sir Harry Lauder, was not his age, but his youth!

He looked young—not so much on the track, but away from the track. One evening during the championships, my wife, Rose, and I visited Liseberg, an outdoor amusement park, and spotted MacLean walking with Australian Cliff Bould, an M65 competitor. They hardly seemed like geriatrics. They strode through the park with a vigor that belied their age. They moved young—and that's something you can't fake. Coloring your hair and removing the bags under your eyes with plastic surgery may give you a surface look of youth, but if you fail to pay attention to what's

> What impressed me about Duncan MacLean was not his age, but his youth!

beneath the surface—your physical fitness—you'll give your age away as soon as you move.

As I continued to compete as a masters runner through the next 3 decades, I used Duncan MacLean as one of my role models. I wanted to be able to move with the same fluidity and still be able to compete when and if I reached his age.

MOVING YOUNG

That probably is part of your motivation, too, as a masters runner, whether or not you might express it in those precise words. And although you may or may not yet have a Duncan MacLean to serve as a role model, physical fitness certainly ranks high on your list of reasons why you run or compete as an athlete. I can say this with some certainty, having surveyed a broad group of masters runners regarding why they ran. In a questionnaire printed both in *National Masters News* and on my Web site, I asked the question: "What is most important to you about running?" The questionnaire suggested eight reasons and then gave the opportunity to provide your own reason.

Among the approximately 500 who responded, nearly everybody (93 percent) chose physical fitness as an important goal. Other categories that respondents considered important were relaxation, camaraderie, and looking good. Only a few (2 percent) were motivated by setting world, national, or other records, but nearly two-thirds of respondents (63 percent) cited setting personal records as important to them.

Regardless of your reason for purchasing this book, I can help you reach your own personal goals. The book is the result of more than a year's intense research and writing, but it might more properly be called the result of a lifetime's pursuit of physical fitness and my own personal love of running as a sport.

Unlike many masters athletes who embraced running as a sport in their thirties—or even in their sixties—I began young. I went out for track my second year in high school for the single purpose of winning a letter. I continued running through and after college, because I realized I was good at it. My peak came at the 1964 Boston Marathon. Despite finishing in fifth place, the first American, I cried, knowing that I probably would never again muster the effort and energy to equal that performance. Time to retire, I thought.

That was 1964. I was 32 years old. I didn't realize that a lifetime of competitive athletics lay ahead of me. The American long-distance running scene at that time was the province of a few hundred dedicated runners, who showed up each year at Boston to test their mettle against the world's best marathoners. Few road races existed outside New England. Few track meets existed for any but student-athletes. Within a year after my fast run at Boston,

WHAT MOTIVATES MASTERS RUNNERS?

Five hundred runners responded to a questionnaire printed in *National Masters News* and posted to my Web site. One of the questions I asked was: "What is most important to you about running?" Respondents were offered the opportunity to choose one or more among eight options. (The numbers below, thus, add up to more than 100 percent.) Here is what motivates masters runners.

Physical fitness	93%
Setting personal records	63%
Relaxation	60%
Looking good	50%
Camaraderie	49%
Competition	21%
World, national, other records	2%
Other	29%

I cut back on my training, content to continue in the sport at a low-ered level of expectation.

At about the same time, a San Diego attorney named David H. R. Pain switched from handball to jogging and thought it might be fun to organize a "masters mile" for the few others his age that he spotted running in Balboa Park. He talked Ken Land, a California promoter, into adding a mile for runners over 40 at a local track meet. The year was 1966. The masters movement had begun! In 1971, having just turned 40, I ran the 10,000 meters and marathon at the first National AAU Masters Track and Field Championships, limited to athletes over that age. So started my second running career.

THE KEY TO CONTINUING

That career continues today, but like the respondents to my ques-tionnaire, I would definitely check physical fitness as the most im-portant reason for continuing into my seventies as at least a somewhat competitive athlete. Personal records? Every time I move into a new 5-year age group, I can set personal records for that age group. Or set single-year age PRs, for that matter. We define our own goals and levels of success. Although I have won four gold medals in world competition, winning another one hardly seems as important to me now. But I both define and refine my goals from year to year, sometimes from month to month. Another World Mas-ters Championships approaches as I write these words, and with a bit more motivation and some additional training, I might not do too badly. Last year, I was ranked ninth in the world in my main event (the steeplechase), and I know I can do better than that.

It is the intent and purpose of this book to make you a better runner. In the pages that follow, I will discuss the running lifestyle and its importance for longevity and overall good health, describing research by doctors such as Ralph S. Paffenbarger Jr., M.D., and Kenneth H. Cooper, M.D., that suggests that by exercising regularly, we can increase our lifespan by 6 to 9 years and improve the quality of that life. I will describe longitudinal research by exercise scien-tists such as Michael L. Pollock, Ph.D., and David L. Costill, Ph.D., who followed the careers of not only elite, but non-elite runners over a period of decades, tracking what health habits allow them to succeed or cause

> Every time I move into a new 5-year age group, I can set personal records for that age group.

them to fail. You will learn how to blend rest and recovery with tough training. All the experts suggest that the best way to improve is to add speedwork to your training, but as a masters athlete, should you do it? And if you cross train, what are the best alternative activities—from cycling to swimming to walking to pumping iron in the gym—that will make you not only a better competitor, but also a healthier individual? We'll also look into the effect of nutrition on performance and how to both prevent and heal the most common injuries plaguing masters runners. I'll offer examples and anecdotes from my own running career and also from the careers of other masters runners. Finally, both at the end of this book and along the way, I'll be offering tips and training schedules for masters runners, men and women. Our needs do differ from those of younger runners.

This is not the first book I have written for older athletes. In 1977, at the start of the first running boom, I wrote *Fitness after Forty,* which landed me an interview on the *Today* show and became a minor bestseller. It was aimed at a somewhat more general audience than a smaller book I wrote later in 1990: *Masters Running Guide.* Published by *National Masters News,* that second book was aimed at a much more specialized audience, those who mostly competed in masters track and field. So much has happened in the sport of running and in the area of longevity since the publication of those first two books that when Rodale asked me if I would like to write an entirely new book aimed at the increasing number of older runners, men and women, interested in improving performance and maintaining good health, I was quick to say yes.

This, then, is that book. I know it will help you achieve your goal, whether that goal is succeeding in competition or living as long (and as well) as Duncan MacLean.

—*Hal Higdon*
Long Beach, Indiana

1 BEGINNINGS

It Is Easy to Improve as a Runner. All You Need to Do Is Start

At the end of my junior year at Carleton College, I traveled to California to compete in the NCAA Track and Field Championships. My focus until that time had been more on getting decent enough grades to graduate and squiring good-looking females to Saturday-night dances rather than in achieving success as an athlete. Thus, it was no surprise that I ran poorly, finishing a nonscoring ninth in the 3000-meter steeplechase. I actually finished last the next day in the 5000 meters. One week later at the National AAU Championships I predictably did no better, placing 15th in a 10,000-meter race that also served as the Olympic trials race for that distance.

Despite such poor performances, I persisted as a runner after graduation in an era when few others did. Why? Because I loved running. I loved to feel the wind in my hair. I loved not only the competitive aspects of the sport, but also the opportunity to socialize with fellow competitors and the solitude running provided: the so-called loneliness of the long-distance runner that those of us who run know is more positive than negative.

And as I continued, I improved. I trained harder, but more important, I trained smarter! Thus, at a period of life when my performances should have begun to deteriorate because of aging, I got better. My confidence in my ability to compete also improved. In

1

my 41st year, I traveled to Europe for a series of masters track meets, "masters" being a separate competitive category for older runners. During a period of 4 days, I ran 3000-meter steeplechase and 5000-meter races at the Crystal Palace Sports Centre in London, England, and a 10,000-meter race in the Olympic Stadium in Helsinki, Finland. I came away with a pair of firsts and one fourth, but more intriguing were my fast times. One was a world masters record; the other two were American masters records. Had I run those same times 2 decades earlier, I would have won one race and placed third in two others at the same NCAA Championships where I had failed so badly as a college junior.

As the years passed, I achieved much more success as a masters runner than I had in high school or college or as an aspiring Olympian. After turning 40, I won four gold medals and five silver and bronze medals at the World Masters Championships. In one of my wins, I set a world M45 record that a quarter-century later remains the American masters record. I also ran more than 100 marathons, the 100th coming at the 100th Boston Marathon in 1996. On my 70th birthday, I set my goal as running seven marathons in 7 months and raising $700,000 for seven separate charities. I not only finished all seven marathons, but more than matched my charity goal.

Thus, if you ask me if you can succeed as a masters runner, I am going to respond with a rousing Yes!

DEFINING SUCCESS

You define your own level of success. It's not necessary to win races and break records to succeed as a masters runner. I've done both, but I take greater pride in the fact that at what to some might be considered an advanced age, I enjoy life. I look good. I feel good. If I no longer run every day, it's because I'm engaged in some other activity, whether swimming or cycling or lifting weights or attending a performance of the Chicago Symphony Orchestra. You can't attend concerts or enjoy other activities unless you're alive—and running keeps me alive. I live to run; I run to live.

Sometimes the bonuses come away from the track. While writing this book, I attended my college's fiftieth reunion. The first evening on campus my wife, Rose, and I attended a reception for the hundred or so of my classmates in attendance and our spouses. One of the women in the class approached to say hello. Her name was Jean. She had been one of the most beautiful women on campus during our 4 years on the Carleton campus in Northfield, Minnesota. And although few sports were offered for women back in that Dark Ages for female athletics, Jean had been an all-state high-school basketball player in Iowa, where girls played that game. Jean and I had dated once or twice, but the competition was pretty tough for this campus queen's attention.

Jean smiled and said to me: "You're better-looking now than you were 50 years ago, Hal." Both our spouses were standing nearby, so I accepted her statement as it was intended: a compliment to my physical fitness. And while I forgot to ask Jean if she was still playing basketball or exercising in some other way, I confess she looked pretty good, too.

Significant scientific research suggests that if we exercise regularly and follow other good health practices, we'll live longer. Epidemiologist Ralph S. Paffenbarger Jr., M.D., of the Stanford University School of Medicine, proved through his study of Harvard University alumni that those who exercised even a minimal amount (gardening, for example) lived more than 2 years longer than those who did not. That was early epidemiological research. With access to more and better data, Kenneth H. Cooper, M.D., founder of the Cooper Institute, the research arm of his medical clinic and fitness center in Dallas, Texas, now suggests that a prudent lifestyle focused on physical fitness might extend life 6 to 9 years! Whether or not we live longer, common sense suggests we can live better by becoming runners. By "better," I mean not having to spend your final years in a nursing home, a burden to your children. A comedian once joked that all

> You can't attend concerts or enjoy other activities unless you're alive—and running can keep you alive.

runners achieve by their frantic exercising is to ensure that they will die in good health. Okay, I'll buy that.

Good health advantages notwithstanding, I know many of you reading these words would like to nibble a few minutes off your 5-K and 10-K times, or maybe even qualify for the Boston Marathon. I'm here to tell you how to do so.

Theoretically, improving performance should prove impossible once you near or pass the age of 40. Although people peak in terms of performance at different points of their life, research with runners suggests that most individuals approach their physical peak in their early twenties and remain near that "best" into their late thirties. After that comes a decline.

According to those who monitor performance, we all should run our fastest 5-K and 10-K times at about age 25. That's when I set

THE 30/30 PLAN

If you are a beginner who never ran a step in your life, you probably need to start gently. And even if you were a track or cross-country runner in school, but haven't run a step in 20 years, you also need to act like a beginner. In fact, you may be more at risk than the newest newbie, because you remember how you used to train and may push too hard too soon.

Here's a simple 30/30 plan to get you going, featuring 30 minutes of exercise for the first 30 days. I'm borrowing it from my own *Beginning Runner's Guide,* a booklet I designed for new runners.

1. Walk out the door and go 15 minutes in one direction, turn around, and return 15 minutes to where you started: 30 minutes total.

2. For the first 10 minutes of your workout, it is obligatory that you walk: No running!

3. For the last 5 minutes of your workout, it is obligatory that you walk: Again, no running!

4. During the middle 15 minutes of the workout, you are free to jog or run—as long as you do so easily and do not push yourself.

personal records for those distances on the track. Ten years later at age 34, I was on the same performance plateau when I ran my fastest marathon time. But 10 years after that, at age 44, I still hadn't lost much. I was that age in Toronto when I won my first World Masters Championships in the 3000-meter steeplechase, my time less than 5 seconds slower than my all-time best from 2 decades before.

I also know masters competitors who achieved peak performances in their forties, fifties, sixties, and even seventies. Norm Green, Paul Heitzman, and Warren Utes come to mind. Of course, they started their running careers later in life, so were able to defeat the decline simply by increasing their training. Warren Utes claims never to have run a step in his life, except to catch the commuter train, until he turned 58. Ten years later, he was still improving while setting age-group records and winning world titles.

5. Here's how to run during those middle 15 minutes: Jog for 30 seconds, walk until you are recovered, jog 30 seconds again. Jog, walk. Jog, walk. Jog, walk.

6. Once comfortable jogging and walking, adopt a 30/30 pattern: jogging 30 seconds, walking 30 seconds, etc.

Follow this 30/30 pattern for 30 days. If you train continuously (every day), you can complete this stage in a month. If you train only every other day, it will take you 2 months. Do what your body tells you. Everyone is different in their ability to adapt to exercise. When you're beginning, it is better to do too little than too much.

In fact, let me offer you an example: Tina Wirth of Jacksonville, Florida, weighed 265 pounds at age 31, when she decided to become a runner. After a period of walking, Tina discovered my 30/30 plan online. Given her weight, it was too tough. Fifteen seconds was all she could run at first. But Tina persevered. Eleven months later and 110 pounds lighter, Tina finished in front of me in the Gate River Run (15-K) in Jacksonville. If Tina can do it, so can you.

If you continue my 30/30 routine for 30 days, you will finish the month able to cover between 1 and 2 miles walking and jogging. That's the first stage in becoming a masters runner.

That raises an impor-
tant point: When you're at
a zero level of fitness, improvement comes easily. I
also must confess that the

> When you're at a zero level of fitness,
> improvement comes easily.

main reason I was able to maintain peak performance over so many
years was that I was a much, much smarter runner at age 44 and
beyond than I was at age 25. One of the goals of this book is to
motivate you to achieve and maintain a higher level of physical
fitness and do so in an intelligent way. Whether or not your goal is
age-group victories and records, I can teach you how to run faster
and live better, too.

SLOWING EQUALLY

That there exist age-group divisions is one reason why masters
runners are able to define their varying levels of success. Every
5 years—as we move from one age group to the next—we are able
to change our goals and remotivate ourselves for success. Masters
competition began in the 1960s when David H. R. Pain, a San Diego
attorney, started a track meet for competitors over the age of 40. Pain
offered separate races in 10-year age divisions, allowing athletes the
opportunity to compete against their age peers. Ten-year divisions
were used to divide competitors at the first World Masters Championships in Toronto, Canada, in 1975, but by the second Worlds in
Gothenburg, Sweden, 2 years later, masters competition had been
subdivided into 5-year groups, as it remains today.

Road running as a participation sport began to emerge at the same
time. The late 1970s featured the start of the first running boom, reportedly inspired by Frank Shorter's victory in the 1972 Olympic
marathon. Frank certainly deserves credit, but a lot of people contributed to the boom, including Arthur Lydiard, Bill Bowerman,
Kenneth H. Cooper, M.D., George Sheehan, M.D., James F. Fixx,
and, yes, David Pain. More and more individuals, mostly males, who
had never participated on their high school track or cross-country
teams, began to enter 10-K races and even marathons. Part of the

growing appeal of road races to people newly fit was the fact that they could earn a trophy or other award for winning or placing high in their age group, even though they did not win the race overall or even come close.

Success had been redefined for masters runners. As we aged, we could continue to remotivate ourselves every fifth year as we advanced into a new age group where we didn't need to be quite as fast as we had in our youth. Everybody else our age was slowing at approximately the same rate, so we remained equals on the starting line, if not the finish line. Canadian Earl W. Fee suggests in his book *How to Be a Champion from 9 to 90* that the secret of success in masters competition is to age more slowly than the other competitors in your age division. Earl had run fast middle-distance times in college, but like many others, he quit competing after graduation to focus on his career. Thirty-three years passed, and he started running again just before turning 55. Within a year after starting back, he set his first world record. Dozens of other world records and titles from the 300 hurdles to the mile followed during the next 2 decades.

Motivation waxes and wanes for many of us. For most of my fifties, I continued to run, but a lot fewer miles than the decade before, while I played around with cross-country skiing and competing in triathlons. Before turning 60, my goals shifted back to my prime sport. I picked up the pace of my training so I could contest for a medal in the steeplechase at the World Masters Championships in Turku, Finland. I was nowhere near as fast as I had been a decade earlier, but I was fast enough to win another gold medal in my new age group.

Jack Foster of New Zealand ran 2:11:19 for the marathon at age 41, winning a silver medal in the Commonwealth Games competing against younger athletes. Foster slowed within the next few decades to a more mortal pace, but nevertheless commented, "I feel like I'm running just as fast as ever—as long as I don't look at my watch."

HOW TO IMPROVE

There are several ways in which you can continue to improve as a masters runner. The easiest and most obvious way is to train harder—or simply start training. If like Warren Utes, you don't start running until age 58, you can begin by running or even walking as little as 1 mile each day. For at least a brief period of time—several weeks, months, or even years—you will begin to improve your level of fitness and be able to run that mile continuously faster even if you do nothing else. Various experts, Joe Henderson among them, have suggested that someone who starts running, almost regardless of age, can continue to improve for 7 to 10 years.

Sooner or later, however, your mile time will plateau, at which point you may need to run farther each day to improve your fitness level: 2 miles, 3 miles, and farther. Even this type of training, how-

---

RUN 2 MILES!

Perhaps the 30/30 plan on page 4 was too easy. Or you've finished that program and want to take the next step. Set as your next goal running continuously for a mile, then 2 miles, then more if you want. The way to do that is to gradually increase the length of time you run in the middle of your workout and decrease the number of walking breaks. Do 45/30 (45 seconds jogging, 30 seconds walking), then 60/30, then 75/30, or 60/15.

Vary your routine. Work a little harder one day, then make the next an easy day. Program occasional rest days when you do no walking and jogging, or cross-training days when you do some other exercise. Test yourself to see if you can run a half-mile continuously, then a mile. It won't happen overnight, but you should begin to see a gradual improvement in your physical fitness.

Here's a 6-week training program for this second phase of conditioning, also from my *Beginning Runner's Guide*. As with the 30/30 training program, begin and end each workout by walking 10 and 5 minutes, respectively. This pattern of warming up, training hard, then cooling down is one used by runners at all levels.

If the above progression seems too difficult for you, either repeat the week you have just completed or drop back to the previous week before continuing. Only you can judge whether you are pushing too fast or too slow, but it's best to err on the conservative side. Also, there's nothing magic

ever, has its limits in the number of miles you can run on a daily or weekly basis. Train too hard, and your times for that mile and other competitive running distances may actually deteriorate.

At that point, improvement will continue only if you learn how to run smarter and realize that the most important workout of any week may be the one defined as "rest." This is true for young runners, but it is even more important for masters runners, who need to train more intelligently than younger runners to achieve success. You need to learn when and how, or even if, to do speedwork and use other training techniques to improve your ability as a runner over and above your base fitness level.

Week	Mon	Tue	Wed	Thu	Fri	Sat	Sun
1	Rest or jog/run	Jog/run 45/30	Jog/run 30/30	Jog/run 45/30	Rest	.5-mi run	30-min walk
2	Rest or jog/run	Jog/run 60/30	Jog/run 30/30	Jog/run 60/30	Rest	.75-mi run	30-min walk
3	Rest or jog/run	Jog/run 75/30	Jog/run 30/30	Jog/run 75/30	Rest	1-mi run	45-min walk
4	Rest or jog/run	Jog/run 45/15	Jog/run 30/30	Jog/run 45/15	Rest	1.25-mi run	45-min walk
5	Rest or jog/run	Jog/run 60/15	Jog/run 30/30	Jog/run 60/15	Rest	1.5-mi run	60-min walk
6	Rest or jog/run	Jog/run 90/30	Jog/run 30/30	Jog/run 90/30	Rest	1.75-mi run	60-min walk

about resting on Mondays or Fridays and doing your long runs on Saturdays. Feel free to adapt this program to fit your own work schedule—although the general pattern and progression should remain about the same. You have taken the next step to becoming a masters runner.

Improvement also may be dependent on a knowledge of how to insert rest, as mentioned above, into your program and when to use alternative activities, such as swimming or biking or even walking, to maintain aerobic capacity. Cross-training does not always work for elite athletes who run twice a day and 120 miles a week to achieve Olympic success, but I can guarantee you that it works for older athletes who have different priorities and abilities.

One of the key longitudinal studies related to the performance of masters athletes was conducted by Michael L. Pollock, Ph.D., who until his death was associated with the human performance laboratory at the University of Florida in Gainesville. Working closely with Dr. Pollock was Larry Mengelkoch, Ph.D., currently an associate professor in the Division of Physical Therapy at Florida A&M University in Tallahassee. While researching this book, I met with Dr. Mengelkoch, and we discussed some of the key points of his late colleague's work. Central to maintaining performance, suggested Dr. Mengelkoch, was volume and intensity. Continue to run the same number of miles and run them with the same degree of intensity, and you will decline very little in performance, not only through your forties, but also through your fifties. It gets tougher after you turn 60, admitted Dr. Mengelkoch.

But nobody said that running, or staying in shape in any sport, was supposed to be easy. Aging is not always fun, unless we do so gracefully. Achieving a high level of performance as a masters runner should always be considered a challenge. I accept it as such, and so should you.

AGING GRACEFULLY

If we did not slow as we aged, there would be no reason for a masters movement. If Sir Roger Bannister still were able to run 4-minute miles in his seventies as he had in his twenties, why establish a separate competitive group in that or any other age category? The fact that the world record for the mile has dropped nearly 20 seconds in the half-century since Bannister first broke the 4-minute barrier begs the question. Runners do get slower as they age. Throwers no longer can throw as far. Jumpers fail to jump as high. The *citius, altius, fortius* motto of the Olympic Games turns backward on us as we move from our thirties

> The secret of success in masters competition is to age more slowly than the other competitors in your age division.

into our forties and fifties, then into our sixties and seventies and beyond. No more is it possible to seek the Olympian goal of faster, higher, stronger. And you don't have to be politically incorrect to note that women move in different orbits than men, their performances almost universally 11 percent slower in events as diverse as the 100 meters and the marathon. As masters statisticians have proved, that's true of women of all ages.

Motivation certainly plays an important part. Sociology also intrudes, because not everybody possesses the wherewithal or the time to train diligently several hours a day. But often we are what we make ourselves. Certainly that was true for me, somewhat of a late bloomer in the world of athletics. Only in my mid-twenties did I begin to realize my potential as a track athlete. A switch to the roads near age 30 failed partly because I did not yet understand what training worked best to run 26 miles 385 yards. Neither did many of my competitors in that era before magazines such as *Runner's World* appeared to serve as both conduits of information and promoters of a growing sport. In a sense, many runners my age were part of a lost generation until the masters movement arrived to offer us motivation to train harder and overcome the failures of our youth. Certainly that was true for the women of my generation, including my female classmates at Carleton, who had relatively few sports activities. The cross-country course on campus passed the large sports field, where women played field hockey in the fall, but after that if you were a woman and wanted some exercise, you had to hope someone asked you to dance. At the first World Masters Championships in Toronto in 1975, only a few women daring enough to admit they were older than 35 appeared. Even today, 3 decades later, women masters competitors lag in numbers behind the men, particularly in the age groups beyond 55.

8 WEEKS TO YOUR FIRST 5-K

In recent years, the 5-K has emerged as America's favorite road racing distance, both for masters and younger runners. One reason is that the 5-K is easily accessible to people just like you, who want to participate in an organized event. Even marathoners like to run 5-Ks as a test of their speed and fitness.

If you're not used to metric measurements, 5-K stands for 5 kilometers, or 5000 meters, or 3.1 miles. Following is an 8-week program from my *Beginning Runner's Guide,* for your third phase of conditioning, culminating with a 5-K race.

After running a 5-K, many runners race no more—or enter organized races only sporadically, maybe once a year. Others run more often, because they enjoy organized competition, even if they have no desire to run fast. Many noncompetitive runners like the carnival atmosphere of races and the camaraderie displayed by other middle-of-the-pack runners. Running races and earning more T-shirts becomes part of their social lives. You can race as often or as little as you like. And you might want to shift from the road to the track and enter a 5000-meter race in a masters track meet. The choice is up to you.

Yet some of my best performances occurred in my mid- to upper forties as motivation and training knowledge merged to allow me to ignore the ravages of time. I ran my second fastest marathon at age 49 while winning a world title in my (M45) age group.

Still, I fully realized that my triumph was temporary. You can fool neither Mother Nature nor Father Time. As I moved into my fifties, I retained the ability to finish first in an occasional local race, but I could no longer stay close in major road races and track meets, unless those events were limited to masters runners. As age caused my times to slow, my motivation diminished somewhat, too. I had been willing to run 100 miles a week to win world titles in my forties, but

Week	Mon	Tue	Wed	Thu	Fri	Sat	Sun
1	Rest or jog/run	1.5-mi run	Rest or jog/run	1.5-mi run	Rest	1.5-mi run	60-min walk
2	Rest or jog/run	1.75-mi run	Rest or jog/run	1.5-mi run	Rest	1.75-mi run	60-min walk
3	Rest or Jog/run	2-mi run	Rest or jog/run	1.5-mi run	Rest	2-mi run	60-min walk
4	Rest or jog/run	2.25-mi run	Rest or jog/run	1.5-mi run	Rest	2.25-mi run	60-min walk
5	Rest or jog/run	2.5-mi run	Rest or jog/run	2-mi run	Rest	2.5-mi run	60-min walk
6	Rest or jog/run	2.75-mi run	Rest or jog/run	2-mi run	Rest	2.75-mi run	60-min walk
7	Rest or jog/run	3-mi run	Rest or jog/run	2-mi run	Rest	3-mi run	60-min walk
8	Rest or jog/run	3-mi run	Rest or jog/run	2-mi run	Rest or jog/run	Rest	5-K race

by my fifties and sixties such effort seemed excessive for someone with a busy life away from running. Priorities change. Also, as I aged and my times inevitably slowed, I realized that more and harder training was not always the answer. It was no longer possible for me to match early-career workouts.

I also had to recognize that decline was an inevitable fact of life. Although no categories existed for masters athletes in the ancient Olympic Games, the Greek philosopher Plato understood that we slowed as we aged. Plato wrote: "Though indeed we may pretend that a person lives and is the same from birth until death, in actual fact he never is exactly in the same condition with the same properties, since everything in him is in a constant state of decay and renewal—his hair, his flesh, his warmth, his blood, and, in short, his whole body; and not only his body, but his soul, his habits, manners and customs, his opinions, wants and desires . . . all are in a constant state of flux, waxing and waning all the time."

THE DECLINE

In *Fitness after Forty* (a book published in 1977 as the masters movement was just getting under way), I described how the human body both developed and deteriorated, beginning with the ovum that begins growing within a mother's womb. In the first few weeks, muscles and connective tissues materialize in the mesoderm; the skin and nervous system develop in the ectoderm; the gastrointestinal tract forms in the endoderm. All through childhood to and after puberty, boys and girls develop into men and women.

"Age 26 is the point—theoretical at least—when the human body has reached its prime," I wrote, "the time at which athletes reach their peak. This point starts the decline, a steady deterioration of the body systems, which eventually results in so-called old age, and death. The slope of the decline is difficult to recognize at first, but it soon turns more steeply downward. It takes a quarter-century for the body to develop its fullest potential, and it takes approximately two more quarter-centuries (according to current actuarial tables) for that body to deteriorate to a point where it no longer functions."

Those words were written when I was 46, when my best performances were behind me. I was suffering from, and confessing to, the inevitable decline that all masters runners must face if we wish to continue in our sport.

"Everyone must slow down sometime," states Joe Henderson, coauthor of *Masters Running and Racing,* "and even if masters runners are still racing as fast as ever, they're probably recovering more slowly."

Aware of this, I am somewhat more sanguine

> At some point, improvement will continue only if you learn how to run smarter.

about my thoughts on decline writing in my seventies than I was writing in my forties. I've learned from experiencing the changes that occur with so-called old age. Yes, we decline, but we decline as masters athletes at a much, much slower rate than we would without the benefits of exercise and good nutritional habits.

"The body continues to develop through life," suggested Jay Berkelheimer, M.D., a pediatrician with the University of Chicago Hospitals. "Although you reach some point in time when all systems start to degenerate, it is arbitrary when that occurs. It probably occurs between 25 and 30 years of life, but there also must be a period when you can maintain your physical capabilities, and that could extend for a long time."

Athletes in different sports seem to mature at different ages, but this may be for sociological reasons as much as physiological reasons.

ESSENTIALS OF SUCCESS

If you want to become a masters runner, here are the essentials for success.

1. **Start to train.** You can't become a masters runner unless you begin. Set a goal for success. Get out and start running today.

2. **Train more.** Almost every training program, whether for the 5-K or the marathon, is based on gradually but consistently increasing the level of stress over a period of weeks and months. Train harder, and you'll run faster.

3. **Train smarter.** Running more and more miles each day in training will only take you so far. You also need to learn how to structure and maximize your training to achieve results.

4. **Learn when to rest.** This is particularly important for masters runners. Taking a day off now and then, or switching to different exercises, will allow you to minimize injuries and thus continue your success.

"Swimmers mature very early," I wrote in *Fitness after Forty*, "reaching top levels in their early teens. Yet few of them continue to improve beyond their

> As I aged and my times inevitably slowed, I realized that more and harder training was not always the answer.

late teens. Sprinters in track achieve peak performances at age 22; milers at age 25; middle-distance runners at age 27; and long-distance runners at age 29. Only rare athletes succeed in Olympic competition into their thirties."

Those words have come back to haunt me, because during the 3 decades since they were written, more and more sprinters have continued to compete at the topmost level of their sport past age 22. Olympic champion Carl Lewis continued to win gold medals into his thirties. Jamaican Merlene Ottey barely lost a step from her sprint speed all through her thirties and ran a remarkable 11.22 for 100 meters at age 43.

A simple explanation exists for this sudden shift in peak performance: money! Beginning in the early 1980s, the organizations that governed the sports of track and field and road running began to allow once-amateur athletes to accept prize money for their victories. (Prior to that time, any money that passed from race directors to athletes was done "under the table.") Motivated by the opportunity to make a living through their athletic ability, runners began to push back the age barriers by training with both greater intensity and intelligence for longer periods of time. This allowed them to prolong the period when they could achieve peak performance, flattening the bell-shaped curve of athletic development and decline.

Nor was improvement limited to Olympic athletes. More "ordinary" athletes found themselves capable of extraordinary achievements. David L. Costill, Ph.D., former director of the Human Performance Laboratory at Ball State University, had middling success as a swimmer while in college at Ohio University, placing 13th in the 200 individual medley at the 1958 National AAU Championships with a time of 2:23.3. While making his mark as a scientist in his twenties and thirties, Dr. Costill ran marathons for competition and recreation. He ran a personal record time of 3:16:32 at age 46, far from the Olympic standard, but good enough to qualify him for the Boston Marathon. Returning to swim competition as a master, Dr. Costill not only bettered his collegiate time with a 2:16.4, but he eventually also won 24 National Masters Championships in a half-dozen different events.

"Our concepts of aging and athletes are going to change," Thomas Bassler, M.D., had predicted in 1977. I quoted Dr. Bassler, a Los Angeles–area physician who was president of the American Medical Joggers Association, when I wrote *Fitness after Forty*. He continued: "We may find out that the peak in performance may be around 29, but the slope afterward is not as steep as we think it may be."

A quarter-century later, Dr. Bassler's words ring truer than ever.

2 AGING

Exercise Scientists Take the Measure of the Masters

I n 1971, 3 days after my 40th birthday, I traveled to San Diego, California to participate in the National AAU Masters Track and Field Championships. Although this was the fourth year for a masters track meet in San Diego under the direction of David H. R. Pain, it was the first year that the growing meet for athletes older than age 40 had achieved sanction from the Amateur Athletic Union as a true national championship.

My motivation might best be described as medium cool. I traveled to the masters meet partly because I had a magazine assignment for *National Geographic* that paid my way to the West Coast. I picked as my main event the 10,000 meters, adding almost as a second thought the marathon. I trained mainly for the shorter-distance event, but not as hard as I would in later years. I figured (somewhat arrogantly), why train hard just to run against a bunch of old men?

The "old man" who served as my main competitor in San Diego was Peter Mundle of Venice, California. As a younger athlete, Mundle had competed for the University of Oregon, whose coach was Bill Bowerman. In fact, Mundle was the first distance runner to achieve much success under Bowerman, a legendary figure who among his many honors served as head coach of the 1972 U.S. Olympic team.

Unlike many runners from his era, Mundle never stopped running or competing after graduation. This gave him an edge at the first Masters Championships in 1968. Just turned 40, Mundle won the 3-mile run at the San Diego meet in 15:15 and the 6-mile run in 31:28. He dominated the distance events in the next two championships that followed in 1969 and 1970.

One of the realities of masters competition, however, is that as you continue, there is always someone younger and faster coming up behind you. At the 1971 meet, I was the new "just-turned-40." While many of the races I have run over a career spanning 7 decades remain little more than numbers in a training diary, I somehow vividly recall the battle Peter Mundle and I waged in the 10,000 at Balboa Stadium, my first race as a master. Peter rushed to the front in the first mile as I confidently let him build up nearly a full-straightaway lead. In the second mile, I stabilized the distance between us and for a time we each moved at the same speed in separate dimensions. In the third mile, I gradually narrowed Peter's lead, eventually pulling up on my rival's shoulder. And for several miles after that, we jockeyed back and forth for the lead, still trading positions going into the last lap. Our finish was furious, but I edged ahead in the final 50 meters, winning in 32:37.9 with Peter only $\frac{3}{10}$ of a second behind. Our final quarter on the 440-yard track was 64.6, faster than I had been able to run a single quarter in practice during the several months leading up to the race.

Runners are funny. Sometimes we take pride from achievements that make no sense to others. I was excited afterward, not because I had beaten Peter Mundle, not because I had won my first National Masters Championships, not because I had run a fairly fast time, but because the two of us had really hammered each other during that last lap. Wow, that was fun! It had brought out the competitive best in both of us. I returned home and spent

Scientists realized that studying human performance could unveil the secrets of how to age gracefully—and perhaps live longer, too.

the rest of the summer working on my sprint speed, peaking with a workout of 3 × 440 with times between 55 and 56 seconds. Judging from my finishing kick, that speed had been there all along. I merely needed motivation to find it.

But he who exalteth himself shall be humbled. Two days after my 10,000 victory, I ran the marathon at the same championship meet. While including a hard race as part of your taper might not have been a decision a sane person should make, I figured that since I had come all the way to California, I might as well get full benefit from my *National Geographic*-paid trip.

As we circled Mission Bay on a multilap course, I eventually positioned myself in front and stayed there past 20 miles, after which my pace slowed. With several miles remaining, a Canadian runner passed and in doing so snarled, "No 64.6 for the last quarter today!" Very rude and probably not very wise, since his put-down might have motivated me to more heroics. Unfortunately, I failed to respond and finished second.

So did my first appearance as a masters runner end in both victory and defeat.

STUDYING HUMAN PERFORMANCE

A more significant encounter at the 1971 National AAU Masters Track and Field Championships in San Diego occurred beside the track with an individual who served as a scientist, not an athlete. Then age 34, Michael L. Pollock, Ph.D., worked as an exercise physiologist at Wake Forest University. In his chosen profession, Mike Pollock was part of a new breed. Although the earliest sports science studies date back to the 1st century and the work of Claudius Galen (a physician who treated gladiators), not until midway through the 20th century did exercise physiology surface as an important scientific discipline. David Bruce Dill, Ph.D., who founded the Harvard Fatigue Laboratory in 1927, is considered by many to be the father of human sports performance in the United States. In the period immediately following World War II, Thomas Cureton, Ph.D., began to achieve status for studies in exercise science with a bright group of

3 × SOMETHING WORKOUTS

When it comes to fine-tuning speed, no better workout exists than 3 × Something. In 1956, I competed in Europe on an American team that included Tom Courtney, who later that year would win the 800 meters at the Olympic Games. Already curious about workouts used by successful runners, I observed Courtney run 3 × 300 meters during a workout in Berlin. Courtney had run 45.8 to win the 440 at the National AAU Track and Field Championships that summer, so he had sprinter speed to complement middle-distance endurance.

But how do you develop speed? Courtney, a Fordham University graduate, began early in the season by running 8 × 330 yards. (American tracks and meets had not yet converted to metric measurements.) He would walk or jog for several minutes between. The speed at which he ran early repeats was probably unimportant; I'm going to suggest he ran around 40 seconds or less. His purpose was to build an early endurance base so he could work on speed later.

As the season progressed, Courtney did fewer repeats rather than more, going from 8 × 330 to 7 × 330 to 6 × 330 to an inevitable 3 × 330. With each numbers drop, he ran faster. Courtney ran in the low 30s the day I observed him.

I modified Courtney's approach, keeping the magic number at 3, but

young students who studied under him. A group of physicians and exercise scientists founded the American College of Sports Medicine in 1954 to share information on both treating athletes and analyzing their performances. From a few dozen individuals in that year, the ACSM has grown now to an organization with 20,000 members in 80 different countries.

"Exercise physiology is the study of how our bodies' structures and functions are altered when we are exposed to acute and chronic bouts of exercise," wrote Jack H. Wilmore, Ph.D., and David L. Costill, Ph.D., in *Physiology of Sport and Exercise.* "Sports physiology further applies the concepts of exercise physiology to training

varying the distance of the repeats. In 1971, I used 3 × 440 to prepare for my 10,000 race against Peter Mundle. Not blessed with sprint speed, I ran 3 × 440 in around 65 seconds before the race. Later that summer, I nudged my repeat times down to 55 to 56 seconds. Two decades later, while coaching the Elston High School track team in my hometown, I used the same 3 × Something approach once a week, with 400 the maximum distance. Run much farther and your focus shifts from speed to endurance.

I varied workouts week to week to avoid having my young runners compare times from one week to the next. I only used the 3 × Something approach at the end of the track season when the weather was warm, with important races approaching. Most important is resting enough so you are fully recovered before starting the next repeat. Usually I walked or jogged the same distance covered in the fast run. Here are some variations.

Number	Distance	Recovery
3	200 m	200 walk/jog
3	300 m	300 walk/jog
3	400 m	400 walk/jog
1 each	400, 300, 200 m	300 walk/jog

the athlete and enhancing the athlete's sports performance. Thus sports physiology is derived from exercise physiology."

Originally, scientists and physicians focused their attention on elite athletes, professional and amateur, because few other than the best continued in competition after graduation from college. In a sense, aerobic sports such as swimming, cycling, running, walking, and particularly the triathlon had not yet been "invented." At the start of the 1960s when I was living on the south side of Chicago and doing my 20-mile-long runs on the weekends along the lakefront as far north as downtown, I would not see another runner. Not a single other runner!

But by the end of the 1960s, the sport of long-distance running began to achieve popularity as an offbeat activity for an increasing number of ordinary people. In that decade, starters in the Boston Marathon, according to Tom Derderian, author of *Boston Marathon,* went from 156 in 1960 to 1,152 in 1969. The goals of these *nouveaux* athletes were more often fun and fitness rather than Olympic medals. Universities took notice and began to add departments where scientists could study athletes, not only those performing in 80,000-seat football stadiums, but those running 10-K races on the roads leading away from those stadiums. David L. Costill, Ph.D., founded the Human Performance Laboratory at Ball State University in 1966. Kenneth H. Cooper, M.D., used the profits from his best-selling book *Aerobics* from 1968 to found The Aerobics Center in Dallas, Texas, focusing his attention on how to utilize exercise to prevent the illnesses of man. Scientists had begun to realize that studying human performance could not only be profitable, but it also could unveil the secrets of how to age gracefully—and perhaps live longer, too. Mike Pollock came along at exactly the right time.

HOW MASTERS AGED

An ambitious young scientist, Dr. Pollock understood that to advance in his profession he would need to embark on a study that not only would improve man's knowledge, but also would be unique enough so that he could attract funds both from his university and the federal government to continue that study and launch others.

As research subjects, Dr. Pollock chose masters athletes, men over the age of 40. He sought to determine how they aged over a period of years; in fact, over a period of decades. Could the fact that these masters participated in competitive sports, and trained at a level that many of their sedentary peers could barely contemplate, improve their physical fitness? Would they live longer? More important: Would they

> The masters runners weren't there merely to run a few laps around the track at a slow pace. They were there to win!

achieve a higher quality of life, at least as measured by standard laboratory tests?

The study proposed by Dr. Pollock could not have been undertaken much before that 1971 track meet in San Diego, because until that time very few athletes continued to compete, much less exercise aggressively, after graduation from high school or college. Only a very, very few in amateur or professional sports continued past the point in life, usually mid-thirties, when they began to slow down. Older people played golf and tennis and skied or bowled, but those were skill sports rather than sports that challenged their muscular and cardiovascular systems. Clarence DeMar won seven Boston Marathons, the last one at age 41, and continued to run Boston until age 65, a few years before his death. But DeMar was an anomaly, the exception that proved the rule that sports were exclusively the domain of youngsters. So was Peter Mundle; and so was I. Until David Pain organized the first Masters Track and Field Championships in 1968, there would have been no masters athletes for Dr. Pollock to study.

Unbeknownst to me when I arrived in San Diego, Dr. Pollock already had begun his study of masters athletes. Identifying several dozen runners who had achieved success in various masters track meets, both national and local, he invited them to his laboratory in North Carolina for a series of tests to measure their aerobic capacity, strength, flexibility, and general physical fitness. Dr. Pollock also asked Jack H. Wilmore, Ph.D., at the University of California in Davis, to assist him in the project. Dr. Wilmore accepted the assignment of testing masters runners who lived west of the Rockies, while Dr. Pollock tested those to the east.

Years later, Dr. Wilmore would recall what impressed him most about the masters runners he saw when he joined Dr. Pollock in San Diego: "Not only were they exceptionally fit for men over 40, but they were intensely competitive. They weren't there merely to run a few laps around the track at a pace slower than they had in high school or college. They were there to win! Or die trying."

One individual at the 1971 meet actually did suffer a heart attack while running the 100-meter dash. Had such incidents occurred with much frequency, it might have blunted the growth of masters competition. But such incidents today seem rare. In the first 15 WMA Championships between 1975 and 2003, only a single athlete would die, according to Torsten Carlius, that organization's president. Ironically, it was an 800-meter competitor who was sitting in the stands watching others compete. Perhaps today's masters runners arrive with a higher level of conditioning. The availability of better physical examinations, including treadmill tests, certainly helps weed out those for whom excessive stress might be risky.

Dr. Wilmore also recalls that he and Dr. Pollock did the study with minimal funding: "The athletes drove or flew to our labs at their own expense. They were eager to be tested and learn as much as they could about human performance."

I failed to receive an invitation, because I had not yet made my mark as a masters runner. For his study, Dr. Pollock had no interest in athletes who might be today's heroes, but would become tomorrow's has-beens. His was a "longitudinal" study, designed to last over a long period of time, in contrast to the majority of sports studies that might last, at best, a few months. Dr. Pollock was more interested in athletes for whom running had at least some chance of being a lifetime habit. He either selected wisely or got lucky in choosing subjects, eventually settling on 27 uniquely motivated individuals, most of whom would continue to compete for several decades.

At some point during the meet in San Diego, Dr. Pollock introduced himself. We discussed the possibility of my being added to his study. For me, as well as for him, it would prove a fortuitous meeting.

Although the other masters athletes had been tested in the spring, a significant body of test data already existed for me in the files of Dr. Costill at Ball State University. When Dave Costill arrived in Muncie in 1966, few distance runners of any distinction lived nearby. Recently moved from Chicago to Long Beach, a small lakefront community in the northwest corner of Indiana, I was the exception. I soon received a call from Dave, who wondered if I would like to participate in a research project of elite marathoners. Others in the study were Boston Marathon champion Amby Burfoot, Olympian Ted Corbitt, and Jim McDonagh of the U.S. Pan American Games team. Curious about what might allow one runner to finish ahead of another, I became a willing participant in that and other scientific studies.

It took 3 hours to drive from Long Beach to Muncie. No expressways connected the two cities. Following directions from Steve Kearney, a training partner who ran on the cross-country team at Ball State, I followed a route that took me through LaPorte, Plymouth, Kokomo, and—my favorite name for a town—Gas City.

Although today's Human Performance Laboratory at Ball State occupies a large 16,000-square-foot building with multiple offices, exercise testing rooms, and access to state-of-the-art indoor and outdoor tracks, when I arrived for my first test in Muncie, Dave Costill operated out of a single room in the basement of the basketball gym. Exercise science got very little respect in this Dark Age. There was barely room for a single treadmill, on the wall in front of which Dave had attached a photograph of a bucolic landscape to give runners being tested something to look at.

Tests performed and measurements made in that era were simple compared to what scientists can do in today's digital age. Most tests centered on the treadmill on which I and others ran for various lengths of time while Dave and his students measured our blood pressure, body temperature, and volumes of oxygen consumed as we breathed into a gas bag. Often tests involved blood being drawn before and after exercise for analysis and, in one instance, Dave stuck a tube down my nose to measure how much fluid still remained unabsorbed in my stomach. At least that was more fun than having your muscles biopsied: Dave or one of his assistants used a needle to slice out a chunk of muscle that could be dissected and viewed under a microscope. The king of biopsied athletes was Ken Sparks, the victim of dozens of biopsies while studying for a doctorate. That didn't seem to slow him down. He ran on a world-record-setting 4 × 880 relay team at the University of Chicago Track Club and later set American masters records from the 800 to the marathon, winning several masters world titles as well.

So began a period when I became a frequent guinea pig in the exercise physiology laboratories of Dr. Costill, Dr. Cooper, Dr. Pollock, and other scientists. Of all the experiments in which I

DRINKING ON THE RUN

Arguably, the single most important sports study of the 20th century was the fluid replacement research performed by David L. Costill, Ph.D., at Ball State University, beginning in the spring of 1968. It benefited not only masters runners, but all runners, fast and slow. As one of Dr. Costill's favorite lab guinea pigs from that era, I was fortunate enough to participate.

The Costill study, funded by Gatorade, sought to determine whether taking water, an electrolyte fluid (guess which one), or both could improve the performance of marathon runners. On 3 successive days, I ran 2-hour runs on a treadmill covering 20 miles each time. One day, I drank no fluids. Another day, I drank water. A third day, I drank Gatorade. Every 5 minutes for the latter two tests, David or one of his assistants would hand me a plastic bottle containing 50 milliliters of water or Gatorade. The fluids went down fine for the first 90 or so minutes, but then that much drinking became almost unbearable. Worse, after the treadmill stopped, David stuffed a tube down my nose so he could pump out my stomach to measure how much fluid I had absorbed.

Other athletes who participated included Amby Burfoot, Ed Winrow, Ted Corbitt, Tom Osler, and Lou Castagnola. We were all in top shape, several of us training for the 1968 Olympic marathon trials. Burfoot, later to become editor of *Runner's World,* won the Boston Marathon that year. Though age 37, I had placed second in the Denver Marathon the month before my test, running 2:35:47 at altitude. Doing 20-mile runs on 3 successive days

participated, however, Dr. Pollock's study of aging masters athletes fascinated me the most and also taught me the most about my own ability to not merely run fast, but also to live long.

MASTERS OF THEIR FATES

While Mike Pollock was able to integrate data from Dave Costill's previous tests, over the next several decades as he moved from Wake Forest to Dr. Cooper's Aerobics Center in Dallas to the Uni-

didn't seem that much a stretch, but with later runners, David decided to program rest days between treadmill runs to make sure everyone finished.

The test proved that by drinking on the run, marathoners could maintain a lower body temperature than if running dry. This translated into a higher level of performance, since when your body temperature soars, you can't run as fast. Much to the dismay of the sponsors, no significant difference existed between plain water and the electrolyte solution in lowering body temperature.

Armed with the results of his tests, David obtained permission from the U.S. Olympic Committee to offer fluids to runners at the Olympic marathon trials later that summer in Alamoso, Colorado, at regular intervals beginning at 5 kilometers, even though international rules in force prohibited aid stations before 15 kilometers. Unfortunately, after the start an official told David that if he offered fluids as planned, any runner accepting aid risked disqualification. I recall running past David near the 5-K point with my hand out. He told me, "Sorry, Hal." I dropped out at 20 miles, one reason being dehydration on a hot and dry day. Although I honestly can't entirely blame the lack of fluids until 15-K, that was partly a factor, both physically and psychologically.

Eventually the weight of Dr. Costill's research caused governing bodies to amend their rules related to fluid replacement. Today, every major marathon offers aid stations early and often. Without fluid replacement, I doubt if the world marathon record would have dropped to 2:04:55 for men and 2:15:25 for women by the time of this writing.

versity of Wisconsin in Milwaukee and ultimately to the University of Florida in Gainesville, Mike continued to test me and the other masters athletes in his longitudinal study.

Twenty-five of the original 27 athletes returned for the 10-year follow-up in 1981. One subject had died in a homicide! Another was not available for testing. Twenty-one remained by the 20-year follow-up in 1991. Among the four more who failed to show, two had orthopedic conditions that prevented them from engaging in regular exercise. Another had Alzheimer's disease. Still another

could not be located, said
Larry Mengelkoch, Ph.D.,
who assisted in the study.

By the 20-year follow-up, the subjects averaged
70 years in age, ranging

> Competition apparently provided the motivation to maintain a more vigorous and healthier lifestyle.

from 60 to 92 years. Having been recruited 3 days after my fortieth
birthday, I was the youngest. After the 10-year follow-up, I had
written a short article on the study for *The Runner* magazine. I noted
that 11 of the 25 continued to compete in masters track meets. Those
11 displayed a significantly higher level of fitness than others who
continued to exercise but not compete. Competition apparently provided the motivation to maintain a more vigorous and healthier
lifestyle. Even more fascinating, I thought, was the fact that three
among the group displayed the highest levels of fitness. I was
among that three. What we did differently was to participate in some
form of strength training. Two of us competed in cross-country ski
races; the third lifted weights. (I did both.) When I pointed this out
to Mike, he commented: "That's not enough numbers to be significant, but I think you're onto something." Ten years later in 1991
when we reported for testing, I discovered that most of those in the
fittest group had picked up on that information and were now in-
corporating some form of strength work in their training schedules.

Disseminating scientific information takes time. Once the scientist has concluded tests in his laboratory, he must analyze the data
and determine the significance of his findings. Often, this involves
consultations with fellow scientists, some of whom may not have
been present for all the tests. Once the scientists achieve consensus
on what they've learned, they begin to disseminate their findings
through the scientific community via publications and at presentations, such as at the ACSM annual meetings.

Since I usually covered those meetings for *Runner's World, American Health,* and other magazines, I often attended presentations by
Dr. Pollock, which invariably attracted a great deal of interest from
his peer scientists. When Mike Pollock first started presenting data
from his longitudinal study of masters runners, he was offered a rel-

atively small meeting room, which proved incapable of holding everybody who wanted to attend. In succeeding years, Dr. Pollock, who served as president of ACSM in 1982–83, often received the largest meeting rooms for his masters running presentation. It was easy to understand why his research was so popular with his scientific peers. Most of them exercised regularly, most frequently by running. They were looking at their own futures.

Dr. Pollock's research was, as the British say, spot-on. Technically,

---

CONVENTIONAL WISDOM FROM WALGREENS

The results from research studies in human performance laboratories about the benefits of exercise now have become part of conventional wisdom: what is now known by all who give the subject much thought. While picking up a prescription at Walgreens, I noticed that the envelope handed me by the pharmacist contained the following advice that seemed to echo words from Mike Pollock's study of aging masters.

Here are some tips on efficient exercise.

- **Aerobic exercise is best for burning calories.** While the recommended 30 minutes of moderate exercise most days helps lower the risk of heart disease and other illnesses, you'll have to push a little harder if you want to lose weight.

- **Exercise harder.** If you simply can't devote 45 minutes a day, 7 days a week to exercise, increase your intensity when you do exercise. People who exercise harder—between 75 and 85 percent of their maximum heart rate—for 20 minutes can burn as many calories as a person walking for 45 minutes.

- **Lift weights.** Resistance training builds bone density, which guards against osteoporosis and builds muscle. You don't have to follow the old three-sets-per-machine formula. Studies consistently show that you can do one set of weight training as long as you progressively lift heavier weights.

Mike also knew how to conduct a study that was clear and precise in its conclusions.

It was nearly a half-dozen years after Dr. Pollock completed his final study of masters athletes until what might be considered the definitive publication of his data appeared in 1997 in the *Journal of Applied Physiology*. Despite 26 years having passed since Dr. Pollock's work began, it was titled "Twenty-year follow-up of aerobic power and body composition of older track athletes" by Michael L. Pollock of the Department of Medicine and Exercise and Sports Sciences, Center for Exercise Science, University of Florida and Geriatric Research, Education and Clinical Center Veterans Affairs Medical Center, Gainesville, Florida. It was coauthored by Larry J. Mengelkoch, James E. Graves, David T. Lowenthal, Marian C. Limacher, Carl Foster, and Jack H. Wilmore. Jack Wilmore later told me that Mike had put Jack's name on the study mainly as an act of professional courtesy, because Jack had not been involved much past the initial testing. "It was Mike's baby," Jack said.

In the opening summary, Pollock et al declare the purpose of their study as to determine the body composition and aerobic power (maximum oxygen uptake, or maximum volume of oxygen, most often referred to as max VO_2) of older athletes after a 20-year follow-up. The testers determined that the 21 subjects remaining in the study divided into three intensity groups, based on their training habits: Nine qualified as high intensity, what might also be referred to as elite. Ten rated moderate intensity. Only two of the 21 ranked as low intensity, showing greatly reduced training.

The testers noted that all groups decreased in maximal oxygen uptake at each testing point. The high group declined by 8 percent of their original max VO_2 by the first 10-year testing, and by 15 percent by the second. The moderate group declined by 13 percent and 14 percent. The low group declined by 18 percent and 34 percent. Maximal heart rate showed a de-

> To maintain fitness, do you run fewer miles, which enables you to run those miles faster, or do you run the same miles, but at a much-reduced pace?

cline of 5 to 7 beats per minute a decade, independent of training status. For the top two groups, body weight remained stable, but body fat percent increased by 2 to 2.5 percent per decade. "Although fat-free weight decreased at each testing point," reported the testers, "there was a trend for those who began weight-training exercise to better maintain it." Leg strength and bone mineral density were maintained from age 60 to 89 for all in the fittest groups, but the weight trainers had a greater arm region bone mineral density than the others.

LIMITING THE DECLINE

Our group of 21 certainly had lost some fitness during the 20-year period, but, according to testers, "less than those shown for the healthy sedentary population." Previous studies indicated that in healthy men, max VO_2 declined by 5 to 15 percent per decade after the age of 20 and through age 75, with the average decline 9 percent. In our more physically active group, the decline was about the same, but because we started at such a high level, we remained much fitter than the healthy sedentary population.

What was the difference in training habits for those within our group? The high-intensity group was identified as those who trained at an intensity between 60 and 85 percent of their maximum heart rates. We also included at least once a week an interval or aerobic threshold training session at 85 percent or higher. In addition, we continued to compete at the top levels, all of us having placed in the top three of a world or national championship the previous year. (I won the M60 steeplechase at the World Masters Championships in Turku, Finland, during the summer of 1991.)

The moderate-intensity group exercised between 60 to 80 percent of maximum, but competed infrequently. Nevertheless, they maintained good health. Compare all in the high and moderate groups to everyone in our age group, the generally healthy population, and we ranked well above the 95th percentile in fitness.

The low-intensity group (keeping in mind that only two remained in this group) exercised up to 70 percent of their maximum, mostly

by walking. They no longer competed. Both were hindered by physical limitations: One had a hip replacement; the other had knee
damage. "It is clear," commented the testers, "that the accelerated
rate of decline in maximum VO_2 (34 percent) between the (10-year
and 20-year follow-ups) was caused by a dramatic reduction in exercise volume and training intensity."

Looking back over the 20 years of the study, our decline had been
slow in the first decade, the miles we trained having remained about
the same. In the second decade, the mileage for all of us lessened,
but more significant: The pace of our training runs dropped consid-
erably. And as both our mileage and the pace we ran those miles declined, so did our maximum oxygen uptake. But what was the cause
and effect? Did we run less and at a slower pace because our max
VO_2 declined, or did our max VO_2 decline because we ran less and
at a slower pace?

I'm going to suggest that it was a combination of both factors. We
were aging, although even the precise numbers determined in the
tests by Dr. Pollock and his peers could not totally unravel all the
causes and effects of that aging process. For myself, I knew that my
slowed training pace forced me to either take a longer time to run
my previous number of miles, or if I limited my workouts to the previous time lengths, I covered fewer miles. Thus the conundrum: In
order to maintain as much fitness as possible, do you run fewer
miles, which enables you to run those miles faster, or do you run the
same miles, but at a much-reduced pace? I'm not sure Pollock et al
can offer me or others the answer to that question. We need to do
both, at least if we want to maintain our edge, if not over our fellow
age-group competitors, then at least over what the testers refer to as
the "generally healthy population." If we continue high-level
training, suggest the testers, we can anticipate that our max VO_2 will
remain much higher than our age peers, "within the 95th percentile
or higher for age-group norms," suggests Dr. Mengelkoch.

"Maximum VO_2 remains relatively constant over time if training
status does not change," reported Pollock et al. When I met with Dr.
Mengelkoch while researching this book, he summarized what he
thought was the most important message of the study. "If you can

maintain the same volume of miles run and the same intensity," said Dr. Mengelkoch, "you will decline very little in your ability as an athlete, at least until about age 60."

Maintain the same volume of miles run and the same intensity, and you will decline very little in your ability as an athlete, at least until about age 60.

Easier said than done, I thought. How, as we age, can we maintain that high a level of training? That is a very, very difficult question to answer. "A critical interaction among age, level of physical activity, and cardiopulmonary function occurs near age 65 to 70," say the testers, "resulting in a nonlinear change in aerobic power." And in another section: "Decreasing levels of physical activity and cardiopulmonary function occurs near age 65 to 70 years, resulting in a nonlinear change in aerobic power."

Dr. Mengelkoch put it more clearly when we talked: "After that age, the physiology of the body changes. What kicks in at that point to diminish the function of the heart and lungs, nobody yet knows." Nevertheless, at least until your sixties, moderate to intensive physical training may allow you to maintain near your peak in performance as a masters runner.

The downside past 60, or any age, is that once you stop training, you gradually lose any edge you had in fitness over others your age, who never ran or trained for any sport. You become what might be described as "average." If you want to remain above average, you need to continue to exercise, even if that exercise is only fitness walking.

Some minor and unexplained differences in decline were shown comparing lower-body and upper-body strength. Lower-body strength remained strong through 89 years, then declined as several members in our group moved into their nineties. But upper-body strength began to decline a decade earlier, at age 79. Does this suggest that runners should focus more attention on strength training for the upper body, beginning when they are younger, or is this merely the natural result in a sport (running) where a relatively low body weight is one prerequisite for success?

In their concluding re-
marks, Pollock et al
stated: "The results
showed that the physical
capacities of older en-
durance athletes declined

"Never get out of shape" should be a
rallying cry for masters runners all
through their lives.

after a 20-year follow-up, even when the intensity of training was
continued at a high or moderate level. A small subgroup who greatly
reduced their intensity of training made substantially larger declines
in physiological capacities and body composition. Body composition changes were related to aging and/or the type of training performed. The inclusion of weight training may be helpful in
maintaining fat-free weight and upper-body strength and bone mineral density with age, but the data from this study are limiting and
do not allow a strong statement concerning this issue."

Because of time delays between the completion of the 20-year
follow-up in 1991 and the ultimate publication of the results by the
American Physiological Society in 1997, the time had passed when
Dr. Pollock might have initiated a logical 25-year follow-up. Seeing
Mike at an ACSM meeting before that 25th anniversary, I asked if
he would be gathering us for more testing. Unfortunately, funding
had become more difficult to secure. Unlike the first year of testing,
few of us would be inclined to jump on a plane and fly to
Gainesville without having our travel expenses covered. Mike said
he hoped that a 30-year follow-up would be possible.

That follow-up would have occurred in the year 2001, when I, the
youngest in the group, turned 70. It did not happen. At the ACSM
meeting in Orlando in 1998, Dr. Pollock presented a paper describing research results on how performing 8 to 12 repetitions (one
set) of an exercise using weights was just as beneficial as performing three sets. It was a classic example of Pollock research that
was spot-on: well-documented to satisfy his colleagues and on a
subject destined to benefit the general public.

Mike also presented new national exercise guidelines, based on a
committee review of published scientific papers. Dr. Pollock had
chaired the ACSM-sponsored group since its inception in 1972.

Alas, before the end of the meeting, Dr. Pollock suffered an aneurysm and died. He was only 61 years old. Unfortunately, the longitudinal study of masters athletes died with him. Nobody, neither at the University of Florida, nor elsewhere in the exercise science community, continued to study those of us whom Mike had recruited at and before the 1971 National AAU Masters Track and Field Championships. How would our group of highly competitive athletes fare as we moved from our seventies into our eighties and perhaps nineties and beyond? The scientific community seems to have lost interest.

HOW TO MAINTAIN YOUR EDGE

Certain truths emerged from the studies of aging athletes by Dr. Pollock and others. Certainly my knowledge of how to maintain good health and top performance as a masters runner has been increased by my participation in Pollock et al. Some important points:

1. **Never get out of shape.** If you already have passed age 35, this news may come late to you. Some children never exercise, and childhood obesity has almost reached epidemic proportions, but most young people become physically inactive and gain weight after graduating from high school or college. Maintaining even a minimum level of fitness through your twenties and thirties will pay dividends later in life. Young women need to begin weight training at this age to limit osteoporosis.

2. **Achieve peak fitness young.** It is easier to create strength and speed in the body when you are younger. Inevitably, every athlete begins to decline in fitness after age 35, but the higher you build your fitness level until that point, the higher a fitness level you should be able to maintain throughout your life.

3. **Intensity is the key.** This is true for all decades, judging from the Pollock study. You don't need to train at the 80 to 90 percent level every day, but including at least one hard (out-of-breath) workout a week can make a remarkable difference in

your general fitness. Interestingly, 71 percent of those responding to my masters running survey indicated that they did some speedwork, indicating the message is getting out.

4. **Rest is as important a factor as intensity.** The Pollock study did not suggest this, but I know from my own training that I cannot train hard 2 or 3 days in a row—or even train hard at all unless my training schedule includes rest, either complete rest or reduced training. Rest is necessary the first day so that you can train hard the second day, and it may be necessary the third or fourth or even fifth day, allowing you to recover so you can continue training at a steady level over an extended period of time.

5. **Easy training also has its place.** Volume of training, the Pollock study suggested, is a major factor in maintaining fitness. If you're a runner, you need those extra miles you accumulate by running a slightly longer distance at least once a week. Short runs or workouts less than an hour are fine most days, but going beyond an hour produces more health dividends. If you can't run longer than an hour as you age, walking may be enough.

6. **Competition can bring out the best in you.** All of us in the high-intensity group remained involved in world, national, or at least local races and championships. It's easier to motivate yourself to train more efficiently, as above, if you have a goal. You don't need to run marathons late in life, but selecting as your goal a half-marathon or 5-K race can provide focus to your training.

7. **Consistency's importance should not be overlooked.** My marathon training programs available on the Internet and in my other books last 18 weeks. But you'll have the most success if you also remain active the other 34 weeks of the year. And while many masters runners crank up their training every fifth year as they move into a new age group, their success is determined as much by what they did the previous 4 years. "Never

get out of shape" should be a rallying cry for masters runners all through their lives.

8. **Don't overlook strength training.** I can't emphasize this enough. While running admittedly is a lower-body activity, your success as a runner depends on your overall health. You can't maintain a healthy body unless you train your upper body, too. It is no coincidence that the most fit individuals in the Pollock study were those of us who did some strength training.

9. **Finally, overall health is important.** You can't continue to compete as a masters runner if you don't stay alive. Regular physical exams every other year, good nutrition, and adequate sleep can help you prevent illnesses that may affect your training and inevitably your overall fitness. You may be able to train through a bad cold, but not the flu, one reason why I get a flu shot every year. Because I am fair-skinned and susceptible to sun damage, I never run without a cap covering my face, plus I also see a dermatologist yearly. Preventive maintenance will help you live longer and run faster.

3 LONGEVITY

Staying Alive Is the Secret for Those Wanting Success as Masters

On one of my visits to Mike Pollock's laboratory at the University of Florida, I flew late one evening into the Orlando airport, renting a car to drive the remaining distance to Gainesville. It was a moonless night, overcast, not a star visible in the blackened sky. I drove along a two-lane highway, pancake flat, through a featureless landscape.

Halfway to Gainesville, my hand accidentally brushed the dashboard light switch, and suddenly the headlights went out. I couldn't see a thing. It was like someone had thrust a canvas bag over my head. Not even another car's headlights in front or behind offered clues to the highway's direction. Only the rumble of tires on concrete signaled that I was still on the pavement.

Momentarily panicked, I fumbled for the light switch but failed to connect. Slowing, I eased the rental car off the concrete and onto a grass shoulder. Stopped, I still could not locate the light switch in the unfamiliar car. I worried that another vehicle might rear-end my unlit car, but no other headlights materialized to light my darkness. I sat helpless as though tied to a chair in a blackened room.

Eventually—but only after what seemed an eternity—I located the light switch and continued my journey, musing about the irony

41

that I might have been involved in a fatal car crash en route to medical tests that could extend my life.

Here's the first secret of masters success: If you want to succeed as a masters runner, you need to live long. If you want to vault from one 5-year age group to another, accumulating trophies and records along the way, you need to survive. Staying alive: That's the secret. Achieving this end, as I discovered on the road to Gainesville, requires a certain amount of luck.

On two previous occasions, I had what might be called near-death encounters. I suspect many of you may have experienced the same. Returning to my Army base in Europe after the 1956 Olympic trials in California, I boarded a bus that drove through a pummeling rainstorm to the airport terminal at Fort Dix, New Jersey. After a wait of several days, I was scheduled on the next departing MATS (Military Air Transport Service) flight to Frankfurt, Germany. Arriving, we were turned back. The flight before mine had crashed, killing everybody aboard. Since the Army randomly assigned passengers to flights depending on when you arrived at the fort, I easily could have been on that airplane.

Several decades later, I drove with my family from Chicago along I-65 to attend the Indianapolis 500, the auto race. Midjourney, I pulled our station wagon off the road so my wife, Rose, could drive. She hadn't been behind the wheel more than a minute when a pair of deer bounded across the highway. Rose braked but still struck one of the deer a glancing blow, killing it and demolishing our radiator and right front fender. We needed repairs to continue, but at least we were uninjured.

I considered the timing of the collision. If we hadn't switched drivers, our car would have been miles down the road when the deer crossed. But had we struck the deer a fraction of a second sooner, it could have flipped through the windshield with who knows what injuries to us and our three children in the back of our station wagon!

Good luck, thus, often rules our destinies and,

> If you want to succeed as a masters runner, you need to live long.

concurrently, our chances to succeed as athletes. A.J. Foyt, an Indy 500 driver, offered what I consider the best comment regarding luck and sports. After a 500 in which another driver's car expired, allowing Foyt to cruise to one of his four Indy victories, the driver shrugged off suggestions by reporters that he had been the recipient of good luck. "Luck," countered Foyt, "is where preparation meets opportunity."

You need a certain amount of luck to succeed as a masters runner. But in many respects, you can control that luck and also increase your chances of living (and competing) to an old age. Mostly, you need to make the right choices.

FINDING GOOD LUCK

"If you want success as a runner," says David L. Costill, Ph.D., "you need to carefully select your parents." Dr. Costill and other exercise scientists have devoted their careers to uncovering the secrets of human performance, but the largest factor determining whether you succeed as a runner—or succeed in any sport from football to basketball to baseball—is genetics. If, like Khalid Khannouchi, you stand 5 feet 5 inches and weigh 125 pounds, you have a greater chance of success as a marathon runner than you do in those other sports just mentioned.

And whether or not you want to call it luck, genetics also affects your longevity. During the summer of 1977, I had breakfast with George Sheehan, M.D., at a Chicago hotel overlooking Lake Michigan. George, then age 59, was in town along with other *Runner's World* contributors, Joe Henderson and Joan Ullyot, M.D., to give a clinic before the first Chicago Distance Classic, a 20-K race. George ordered bacon and eggs, and I chided him for ordering what some cardiologists might consider an "unhealthy" meal, containing an excess of fats and protein.

"You need to know what killed your parents and grandparents," George defended his meal choice. "If your parents died of heart attacks, you wouldn't order this breakfast. But most of the people in my family die of cancer, and that's probably what will kill me."

George proved to be a prophet. He died in 1993 of prostate cancer a few days short of his 75th birthday—although he did survive 7 years after first being diagnosed with that disease. His healthy habits probably helped George lengthen his life and certainly allowed him to enjoy it more until the end. By that time, he had modified his eating habits, because continuing research had begun to suggest that good nutrition might improve your ability to avoid cancer and many other diseases—or at least postpone the end.

Certain strategies can help you do just that. The good news for masters runners is that the strategy that promises the most health benefits, including longest life, is what we all love to do best: exercise. Not only that, but the best exercise is (drum roll, please) running! Epidemiologists, those scientists who use statistics in their search for knowledge, have begun to offer overwhelming evidence that exercise can provide us with the Fountain of Youth that Ponce de León sought but failed to find.

LINKING EXERCISE AND LONGEVITY

Among the scientists who seek to provide a link between exercise and longevity is Ralph S. Paffenbarger Jr., M.D., professor of epidemiology at Stanford University School of Medicine. In 1988, Dr. Paffenbarger was invited to deliver the prestigious J.B. Wolffe Memorial Lecture at the annual meeting of the American College of Sports Medicine in Dallas. I was in the packed auditorium. At the start of the lecture, he provided a concise definition of his own profession: "Epidemiology is the study of frequencies and distributions of disease in human populations that can be described in terms of time, place, and personal characteristics to establish (1) the cause of a disease, (2) the means of its spread, and (3) a mechanism for surveillance of its occurrence. To accomplish these purposes, epidemiology requires the application of clinical knowledge, inductive reasoning, statistical methods, scholarly logic, and common sense."

Of those methods, Dr. Paffenbarger suggests that common sense may be most important for any scientist achieving success in his profession. I have known Ralph Paffenbarger for many years, seeing him most often at parties given in the home of Jack H. Scaff Jr., M.D., founder of the Honolulu Marathon, before that race, which we both usually ran. "Paff," as his friends

> The good news for masters runners is that the strategy that promises the most health benefits is what we all love to do best: exercise.

know him, had a distinguished career as a long-distance runner, running 151 marathons with a career best of 2:44:39 at a marathon in California's Napa Valley in 1971 at age 49, a remarkable performance. He also ran ultramarathons, including the London to Brighton Marathon in England and the Comrades Marathon in South Africa, both races of near 54 miles. One year, Paff ran the London Marathon on a Sunday, the Boston Marathon on a Monday, and the Jersey City Marathon the following Saturday. "An absolutely ridiculous thing to do," he laughs about the feat now. Paff's last marathon was in 1993 at Honolulu. He walked the race in 7:13:39 at the age of 71.

Ralph Paffenbarger, however, will be remembered less for his skills as a long-distance runner and more for having conducted what many consider the mother of all longevity studies, that of Harvard University alumni and their exercise habits. Interestingly, Paff made his mark as a scientist by working for one university (Stanford) and studying the alumni of another university (Harvard) on opposite ends of the United States. He chose Harvard only after considering a number of universities. "Harvard had the best data on the health of its alumni," Paff explains.

While discussing the Harvard alumni in the Wolffe Lecture, Dr. Paffenbarger also summarized several earlier studies of British civil servants, San Francisco longshoremen, and Iowa farmers. In 1953, Professor Jeremy N. Morris of London matched sedentary drivers of London double-deck buses with their physically more active conductors, whose duties required them to continuously go up and down stairs. "The conductors had significantly less coronary heart disease," reported Dr. Paffenbarger. "What disease they had was less severe, and they were more likely to withstand an attack than were the drivers. Morris et al checked and discarded many other explanations before concluding that this was due to differences in energy expenditure on the job. Today we would conclude also that the conductors were physically more fit than were the drivers."

The same appeared true of San Francisco longshoremen, those who worked on the docks versus those who worked cushier jobs in the office. The study involved 6,351 longshoremen over a period of 22 years between 1951 and 1972. Those who were cargo handlers did very heavy work loading and unloading shipments in the holds of big oceangoing vessels—pulling, pushing, shoving, lifting, heaving, and shoveling, mostly by might and main. When these tasks were translated into their energy expenditure demands, the men in jobs requiring 8,500 kilocalories or more per week were found to have much lower risks of fatal coronary heart disease than were men who held less-demanding jobs, such as tally clerks, hoist operators, and foremen.

Translating that many kilocalories, as spoken of by scientists, into calories, as recognized by the general public (see "Calories vs. Kilocalories," on page 47), and then into running terms, you would need to run close to 85 miles a week to burn 8,500 calories. That's a lot of running and a lot of calories burned. To put that in context, Tour de France cyclists burn even more calories and in a shorter period of time. Tour cyclists typically cover 100 miles a day, burning an average of 6,100 calories daily while on their bicycles and approximately 8,000 total calories a day through all activities. The highest single day as reported in a study of four Tour cyclists published in the *International Journal of Sports Medicine* was 7,800 calories on the bike, probably near 10,000 calories for all activities. Although it took the longshoremen a week to burn as many calories as a Tour cyclist might in a single day, 8,500 calories is a massive amount for anyone to burn in their job-related activities.

One of the requirements for an outdoor longshoreman getting an office job indoors was at least 5 years having worked in the more physically active job outdoors. Those studied averaged 13 years of outdoor work before moving inside. Dr. Paffenbarger suggested this ruled out the possibility of "self-selection," meaning the sedentary

CALORIES VS. KILOCALORIES

In measuring energy expenditure, scientists use the term kilocalories, what seemingly would be a thousand calories. A calorie, according to *The Random House Dictionary of the English Language,* is "an amount of heat exactly equal to 4.1840 joules." I won't even attempt to explain "joules," because I can see that I've already lost you.

For, as a matter of fact, the general public does not understand "kilocalories." We only understand the calories that we see on the labels of food and read about in diet books. We are more used to the term "calories" without the "kilo," which often gives scientists pause. When we want to lose weight, we are content to burn calories and don't want to hear anyone confuse us by suggesting we actually are burning kilocalories.

"This started with nutritionists using 'Calorie' with a capital 'C' to mean a kilocalorie and using 'calorie' with a lowercase 'c' when they were talking to the general public," explains David P. Swain, Ph.D., a professor of exercise science at Old Dominion University. "Later, the nutritionists stopped bothering to capitalize the word calorie and left us with having to call 1,000 calories a calorie."

Dr. Swain smiles as he continues: "It would be the same as if I told you I weighed 142 ounces. They're really pounds, but who cares?"

It is a generally accepted fact that a runner of average weight, meaning 150 pounds, burns 100 calories for every mile he runs. That's not entirely true either, but a scientist would suggest that the runner actually burns 100 kilocalories, or 100,000 true calories, the kind that are equal to 418,400 joules. Stop rolling your eyes; I'm almost finished!

To avoid confusion, in this book, when I speak of calories I mean the calories recognized most often by nutritionists and the general public. I figure the scientists are smart enough to translate calories into kilocalories in their minds.

men did not engage in physical activities because they were unfit or already had impaired cardiac function.

About longshoreman longevity, Dr. Paffenbarger reported: "Sudden-death heart attacks were less common among the cargo handlers (compared to office workers) either because they had fewer heart attacks or because they were better able to withstand them."

IOWA FARMERS ARE FIT, TOO

Similar conclusions occurred from a comparison of Iowa farmers with townspeople. A study headed by P. R. Pomrehn published in the *Journal of the American Medical Association* in 1982 looked at 62,000 deaths among Iowa men ages 20 to 64 from 1962 through 1978, focusing on 95 farmers and 158 townsmen. The physically active farmers had 10 percent lower coronary heart disease risk than nonfarmers. "The farmers," summarized Dr. Paffenbarger, "had higher caloric intake and higher blood cholesterol levels and slightly higher body-mass indices, but were less obese by skin-fold test, and their frequencies of cigarette use and alcohol consumption were less than half those of nonfarmers. The farmers were twice as likely to be physically active and were more fit by treadmill test as contrasted with nonfarmers."

Following up on his study of London bus drivers and conductors, Professor Morris later studied the lifestyle and health of 17,944 civil servants, whose desk-work assignments, said Dr. Paffenbarger, "deprived them of virtually any vigorous physical activity on the job. But some of these Britishers were habitually brisk about their household duties, gardening, and recreational sports play after work and on holidays. Those who enjoyed vigorous yard work, hiking, running, and sturdy games had a coronary heart disease incidence half as high as that of their fellow workers who were less active in their leisure time."

One conclusion reported by Morris and echoed by Dr. Paffenbarger should prove particularly interesting to those masters runners who include in their training speedwork, strength training, or other exercises that force their heart rate above the "conversational" 65 to 75 percent of maximum. "The strongest evidence of a protective effect," said Dr. Paffenbarger, "pointed to intensity of exercise rather than totals of all physical activity whether light or strenuous. . . . Men reporting eight or more sports-play episodes in 4 weeks (or at least twice a week) had only 36 percent of the coronary heart disease risk of men who played no sports at all."

All this served as prelude to Dr. Paffenbarger's own landmark research on Harvard alumni, begun in 1960. The 16,936 individuals included in the study entered Harvard University between the years 1916 and 1950. "The extensive information we have on these men," reported Dr. Paffenbarger in the Wolffe lecture, "has been gathered from university archives recorded in their student days, from successive sets of mail questionnaires completed by the alumni in their years of middle life or old age, and from official death certificates of those classmates who passed away. Thanks to the cooperation of the university alumni office, hardly a fraction of 1 percent of these alumni has been lost to follow-up for mortality, while up to 70 or 80 percent of the living have loyally returned a succession of personal questionnaires for study."

In 1972, 10 years after the first data collection, Dr. Paffenbarger noted that 572 individuals experienced "first clinical attacks of coronary heart disease." By 1978, there had been 1,413 all-cause deaths, 441 from coronary heart disease. Also available for study—and the key to its conclusions—were the exercise habits of Harvard alumni, whether they walked, climbed stairs, or engaged in other recreational pursuits that burned calories. The Harvard records also included whether or not their alumni had participated in intercollegiate sports during their years on campus. Whether they had or had not been "jocks" apparently provided no protection against heart attacks. What counted was whether they continued, or began, to exercise. The numbers showed that alumni who expended 2,000 or more calories a week exercising had

> College laggards who became physically active as alumni achieved the same benefits as their classmates who had been active all along.

39 percent lower risk of coronary heart disease than their less-active classmates. "College laggards who became physically active as alumni achieved the same benefits as their classmates who had been active all along," reported Dr. Paffenbarger.

A published version of Dr. Paffenbarger's Wolffe Lecture included a chart that showed the benefits gained by burning more than 2,000 calories a week through exercise. Seemingly, this would mean that you would need to walk or run 20 miles a week, but Dr. Paffenbarger also included what might be called "side" exercises, such as walking up stairs or working in the garden, that you would do in addition to a planned exercise, such as walking or running. Fewer died among those burning 2,000 calories or more through exercise than those who exercised less, their rate of coronary heart disease was less, and their risk was 61 percent that of their more sedentary classmates.

Also studied was the "dose-response" relationship between increasing energy expenditure and decreasing coronary heart disease incidence. Risk declined as energy output increased from less than 100 to 3,500 calories a week. While gardening and walking helped decrease risk, the biggest benefits came when the energy expenditure represented "vigorous sports play," which included running. "Apparently the dose-response relationship of exercise versus coronary heart disease," reported Dr. Paffenbarger, "was not merely a matter of total energy output per week but also reflected *intensity* of exercise."

The message was simple: Fail to exercise, and die young. Dr. Paffenbarger comments further: "In the case of physical activity and heart disease, it's not the fact that someone didn't exercise last week that may cause a heart attack this week; rather, it is a habitual pattern of inactivity over a period of months, years, or decades that appears to relate to disease."

More intriguing to those of us who like to attract readers by writing catchy headlines, Dr. Paffenbarger was able to determine from

> The message was simple: Fail to exercise, and die young.

WALKING VS. RUNNING

Regardless of whether you exercise by walking or running, you burn the same number of calories for every mile you cover. Right? Most exercise charts suggest that a walker weighing an average 150 pounds burns 100 calories a mile, and so does a runner. That's because you're pushing the same number of pounds over an equal distance. Can that be true?

David P. Swain, Ph.D., brands that as an urban legend. The error, he says, comes in totaling calories burned (resting needs plus exercise needs) during the length of the walk or run. "Since the walker takes a lot longer," Dr. Swain explains, "she utilizes a higher number of calories from resting needs over the longer time period. But walking itself is more efficient than running, and the average-size person only burns an extra 50 calories for 1 mile of walking, versus 100 calories for 1 mile of running." Only the net (exercise-induced) calories burned should be counted when looking at the benefits of exercise, suggests Dr. Swain.

"If you want to lose weight," he adds, "it takes twice as many miles of walking as running to burn the same number of calories." For reducing heart disease risk, it probably takes more than twice, because, as Dr. Paffenbarger points out, it's not just the calories you burn, but the intensity at which you burn them.

the data on Harvard alumni how exercise significantly improved their longevity. The evidence was clear: Exercise now and you would live more than 2 years longer. The average longevity gain for alumni ages 35 through 79 was 2.15 years, but how much longer you lived depended partly on when you began to exercise. Someone who began to exercise at age 35 could extend his life 2.51 years. Wait until age 75 to begin, and you still can expect to live 0.42 year longer, much less than had you started earlier, but those extra 5 or so months of life still could be precious. Dr. Paffenbarger's figures are listed on page 52.

The Harvard alumni data also suggested that there is no time lost to exercise. People often use as an excuse not to exercise, "I don't

Start to exercise at age . . .	Years of life gained
35–39	2.51
40–44	2.34
45–49	2.10
50–54	2.11
55–59	2.02
60–64	1.75
65–69	1.35
70–74	0.72
75–79	0.42
All ages: 35–79	2.15 (average)

have time." Actually they would save time. Depending on how vigorously you exercise, you get anywhere from an hour or two of extra life for every hour you exercise.

"Moreover," concluded Dr. Paffenbarger, "these extra hours would very likely be added into the vigorous mainstream of (your) life experience, not spent confined in a wheelchair or rest home as an aged invalid."

You apparently also can control your longevity by the amount of energy you expend in exercise. While 2,000 calories provided an interesting point for dividing the fit from the less fit, further subdividing the Harvard alumni into how many calories they burned a week provided additional evidence that, at least to a point, the more they exercised, the less their risk of heart attack. Among those whose physical activity was less than 500 weekly calories burned, the number of deaths per 10,000 worker-years was 93.7, which in the study was assigned a relative-risk-of-death index of 1.0. As calorie burn increased in weekly dosage, deaths decreased to 42.7, the risk therefore declining to a statistical 46 percent. Here are Dr. Paffenbarger's figures, as published in 1990 in a book titled *Exercise, Fitness, and Health.*

Most of us would settle for 2 more years of life as a beneficial

Calories burned/week	Deaths/10,000 worker-years	Risk
<500	93.7	1.00
500–999	73.5	0.78
1,000–1,499	68.2	0.73
1,500–1,999	59.3	0.63
2,000–2,499	57.7	0.62
2,500–2,999	48.5	0.52
3,000–3,444	42.7	0.40

side effect of being a masters runner, but subsequent work by other researchers suggested that, if anything, Dr. Paffenbarger may have been conservative in his projections. He admits this, too. This was necessary because as an epidemiological researcher using the records of Harvard alumni, living and dead, he was dealing with numbers as much as people. Just as studies of London bus drivers, San Francisco longshoremen, and Iowa farmers inspired Dr. Paffenbarger in his study of the Harvard alumni, he would inspire the next generation of epidemiologists. That would include people in the employ of best-selling author and exercise guru Dr. Ken Cooper.

KEN COOPER'S PATIENTS

Soon after founding the Aerobics Center and its associated Cooper Clinic in Dallas, Kenneth H. Cooper, M.D., began accumulating the records of patients. As Dr. Cooper's books continued to sell and as people began to flock to his Center and Clinic, Dr. Cooper invested some of the profits in a research branch: the Cooper Institute, currently directed by Stephen N. Blair, P.E.D.

Harvard alumni who expended 2,000 or more calories a week exercising had 39 percent lower risk of coronary heart disease than their less-active classmates.

HOW MUCH INTENSITY?

Research on individuals enrolled in the Harvard Alumni Health Study continues with I-Min Lee, M.D., associate professor of medicine at Harvard Medical School. (Dr. Paffenbarger, she insists, remains fully involved in reviewing data.) While earlier analysis suggested that burning 2,000 calories a week through various forms of exercise promoted longevity, how intense must that exercise be?

Dr. Lee followed 7,337 men with an average age of 66 over a period of 5 years. On first contact, she asked them to use perceived exertion to rate the intensity of their exercise. Eight percent rated their exercise level as weak, 27 percent strong, with most in the middle.

At the 5-year follow-up, Dr. Lee discovered that 551 of the men had developed coronary heart disease. Those who exercised more intensely were much less likely to contract the disease.

Like Dr. Paffenbarger, Dr. Blair enjoyed long-distance running, having run 17 marathons and one 50-mile ultra with a marathon best of 3:28:22. (Coincidentally, both Dr. Paffenbarger and Dr. Blair achieved their personal records in Napa Valley, California.) Dr. Blair also shared Dr. Paffenbarger's interest in numbers and the effect that exercise had on physical fitness and longevity.

Dr. Blair first started traveling to Dallas to provide assistance as a researcher for Dr. Cooper in 1980 while still a professor in the School of Public Health at the University of South Carolina in Columbia. In 1984, he joined the Cooper staff full time and began to focus on the large body of information available about patients who received physical examinations at the Cooper Clinic beginning in 1970.

As a friend of Ken Cooper, I was one of those patients. Ken had been high-school state mile champion in Oklahoma and later ran the 4 × 880-yard relay for the University of Oklahoma before attending medical school. Graduating, he joined the U.S. Air Force, one of his assignments while stationed in San Antonio, Texas, being to determine how astronauts could maintain their physical fitness while

Exercise rating	Percentage	Lessened risk
Weak	8%	0%
Moderate	39%	19%
Somewhat strong	27%	38%
Strong or more intense	27%	40%

Interestingly, there seemed to be little difference in protection (38% versus 40%) between those who rated their exercise as somewhat strong and those who exercised more intensely. This suggests that you have to train hard to diminish your chances of suffering from coronary heart disease, but you don't need to train too hard.

coping with the weightlessness of space. That quest led to a point system for exercise eventually translated into his best-selling book, *Aerobics*.

His college track days behind him, Ken nevertheless continued to jog for enjoyment and because he sensed that it would improve his health—although he did not yet have proof that this might be true. I first encountered Ken when he ran the Boston Marathon in 1962 and 1963. The Air Force had sent Ken to Harvard for a graduate degree, and he began training with two friends of mine: Warren Guild, M.D., the medical director of the Boston Marathon, and John J. Kelley, two-time winner of that race who ran Boston a record 61 times. More half-miler than marathoner, Ken struggled in the last half-dozen miles. He was the last recorded finisher in 1962 with a time of 3:54 in 101st place, but trained harder and improved that time by nearly 40 minutes the following year. Ironically, he improved by only two places to 99th. Running was about to emerge as a mainstream sport. In 1962, only 181 started the Boston Marathon; 1 year later, the number was 285; and a year later, after an article I wrote about Boston titled "On the Run from Dogs and People" appeared in *Sports Illustrated,* a record 369 entered. We did not realize it at that time, but the running boom was about to begin.

With the publication of *Aerobics* in 1968, Ken Cooper became an important promoter of running in the combined role of celebrity speaking to the masses and as a source of information about the relationship of exercise to fitness and longevity. I interviewed Dr. Cooper in 1968 for a *New York Times Magazine* article about the growing popularity of jogging. At a medical conference at the University of Nebraska several years later, I happened to sit beside Ken during one of the lectures. He tapped me on the shoulder and said, "Your pulse rate is 29."

One of the secrets of my success as a long-distance runner is a strong cardiovascular system, a "big heart." I also possessed what once was considered an abnormally low pulse rate. (The Red Cross refused to allow me to donate blood in college.) But it puzzled me that Ken knew my pulse rate.

Ken smiled and pointed to my crossed leg and raised trouser, which had exposed to view a pulsing artery. "I counted," he smiled.

About that same time, I began to make regular visits to Ken's office in North Dallas because of various magazine assignments. In a chapter about Dr. Cooper in my 1977 book, *Fitness after Forty,* I described his growing complex of Colonial-style buildings in North Dallas as "a Disneyland for joggers." The main building featured a fitness center with lockers, indoor exercise equipment, a gymnasium, and an outdoor pool and tennis courts. Next door was the Cooper Clinic, where Dr. Cooper and a growing staff of physicians examined patients. Eventually he added a guest lodge and a separate building for his research arm, the Cooper Institute. A mile-long, rubber-surface jogging track circled the grounds, and if you came by late in the afternoon, you might spot Ken himself doing his regular 2 or 3 daily miles. No longer a competitive runner, Ken claims that (based on his research) if you run more than 15 miles a week, you're doing it for reasons other than fitness. Some veteran runners object to this statement as disparaging, but I agree with his point. Many of us run for fun or competition; fitness comes only as a by-product, a positive side effect.

Dr. Ken Cooper claims that if you run more than 15 miles a week, you're doing it for reasons other than fitness.

My research as a writer led me to realize that regardless of how many miles a week you run or how well you eat, and even if you never have smoked cigarettes or committed other crimes of the body that normally impact longevity, you still need regular physical examinations to detect oncoming problems if you want to live long. Even nonsmokers can contract lung cancer from secondhand smoke. Diseases such as diabetes, while they can be controlled by exercise, often are a result of hereditary influences. I began to get regular physical exams at the Cooper Clinic, urging my wife to do the same.

The physical exams were complete and lasted most of a day. Normally, Rose and I fly into Dallas the afternoon before an exam and check into the guest lodge on the grounds, eating at a nearby restaurant but avoiding a glass of wine, since no alcohol is permitted 24 hours before the blood tests. Although tests include everything from body fat composition to hearing and eyesight, the key element remains the exercise stress test where you run (or walk) on a treadmill until you can go no farther. If you have coronary heart disease, it should be apparent from your blood pressure and electrocardiogram measurements.

One such visit I made to the Cooper Clinic occurred in 1984, not too long after James F. Fixx, author of the best-selling *The Complete Book of Running,* died of a heart attack while running. The previous fall, Fixx had visited the Cooper Clinic not for a physical exam, but to observe marathoner John J. Kelley running on a treadmill, an assignment for *The Runner* magazine. "I offered to test Jim for no charge," Ken later told me, "but for whatever reason, he declined. If Jim had agreed to be tested, he might still be alive today."

That same year, Steve Blair moved to Dallas to work full time for the Cooper Institute and began to direct his attention to the mass of patient data available to him. With an eventual 18 physicians seeing a half-dozen patients a day, information on the physical fitness of patients accumulates like ice on the lip of a glacier. To date, Dr. Blair has data on 80,000 patients, some of whom exercise, some of whom do not. Over a period of years, Dr. Blair and his colleagues have begun to sift through this data to determine what lessons they can learn.

A DEPTH OF DATA

If there is one difference between the Harvard studies and the Cooper studies, it is the availability of a greater depth of data involving people seen in person, including the results of treadmill (stress) tests, blood pressure and body fat measurements, blood lipid profiles, and tests involving various other benchmarks of fitness. The result is that Dr. Blair has helped reinforce the studies of London bus drivers, San Francisco longshoremen, Iowa farmers, and Harvard alumni.

Yes, exercise will improve your physical fitness and permit you to live a longer life.

In proving this to be true, Dr. Blair first divided his subjects into five fitness groups from low fit to high fit, but eventually narrowed this to three groups, calling the group in between moderately fit. According to Dr. Blair: "The biggest health benefits come if you can move from low fit, where you do almost no exercise, to moderately fit, where you do at least some exercise. If so, you can cut by 50 percent your risk of having a heart attack."

How much exercise? Dr. Blair suggests 140 to 150 minutes of walking a week. In other words, walk for a half-hour, 5 days a week. Jogging 90 minutes a week, he says, would achieve the same end. Someone walking at a brisk 15:00-mile pace for 150 minutes or jogging at 9:00-mile pace for 90 minutes would cover nearly 10 miles

> If Jim Fixx had agreed to be tested, he might still be alive today.

and burn approximately 1,000 calories. That is about how far I walk each morning while staying in our winter condominium home in Florida. Before breakfast, I stroll to a nearby gasoline station to purchase a copy of the *Florida Times-Union*. Depending on which route chosen, I cover between 1.5 and 2 miles. Most people without physical disabilities could do the same and burn 1,000 calories, meeting Dr. Blair's criteria for becoming moderately fit. Of course, the problem is that most people do not choose to exercise even this minimum amount.

I choose to do more, mostly running at low tide on the Atlantic Ocean beach near our condo or lifting weights or swimming laps at a fitness center I pass on the way to the beach. (Yes, I chose to buy that particular condo partly because of its easy access to the beach and good exercise facilities.) I easily burn another 1,000 calories a week, which by Dr. Blair's definition, raises me to the level of high fit. The decrease in risk is only another 15 percent, but you add years to your life.

How many years is another question, and although Dr. Blair and Dr. Paffenbarger both know the answer, they hesitate to state numbers. The "common sense" that Dr. Paffenbarger mentioned in his Wolffe lecture is not enough proof. To meet the test of science, epidemiologists not only need to do the research, but they need to present their findings to their peers for review before publication in scientific journals, at which point their colleagues can agree whether they are right or wrong. That being the case, you can accept as fact or fiction the suggestion that if you move from low fit to moderately fit, you can live for an additional 6 years. You can choose to deny or agree that moving from moderately fit to high fit will add another 3 years to your life, a total of 9 years extended longevity. Dr. Paffenbarger's earlier research with the Harvard alumni had suggested about 2 years of added longevity. In a private conversation recently, he suggested that by exercising either steadily or vigorously or both, you may be able to increase your lifespan 7 to 10 years. Is that science or common sense?

In an interview published in the January 1999 issue of *Nutrition*

SEEKING LONGER LIFE

Ponce de León sought the Fountain of Youth and failed to find it. Scientists since then have sought ways and means to extend life—or at least prove that life *can* be extended. Exercise combined with a healthy lifestyle seems to offer the best means of both extending life and providing for a higher quality of life. "Exercise can help you live longer and make you less likely to die of heart disease and stroke," states Steven N. Blair, P.E.D., of the Cooper Institute, in an interview published in the *Nutrition Action Healthletter,* January 1999. "It can reduce the risk of type 2 (adult-onset) diabetes and colon cancer. And almost everyone believes that an active life should prevent obesity, though that hasn't been studied in detail."

But how much longer? And how active a life? How many miles a day must we run in the footsteps of Ponce de León? In his study of the Harvard alumni, Ralph S. Paffenbarger Jr., M.D., suggested that someone age 35 who exercised enough to burn an extra 2,000 calories weekly might enjoy 2.51 extra years of life. In the *Healthletter* interview, Dr. Blair suggested 2 to 3 years of extra life. Privately, however, scientists suggest that it may be possible to better those numbers. Kenneth H. Cooper, M.D., told me people could live 6 to 8 years longer with proper doses of exercise. Dr. Blair

Action Healthletter, Dr. Blair used the more conservative, but accepted, estimate of 2 or 3 years. "That doesn't seem like very much," commented Dr. Blair, "but if someone tomorrow found a magic bullet that completely cured all cancer, average longevity would increase by a bit more than 2 years."

VICTIMS OF THEIR GENERATION

I thought of my father, the last time I had seen him alive. "Hig" (as his friends all called him) was just a month short of his 70th birthday, lying in a hospital bed, an oxygen mask on his face so he couldn't talk, tubes coming from his arm, a very frightened look on

amended that number in another conversation to 6 to 9 years. Dr. Paffen-barger mentioned 7 to 10 years, also in a private conversation. But scientists don't always want to confirm longevity data publicly until their research studies are published and peer-reviewed.

The following chart is based not on the work or words of any one scientist, but rather on conversations with many of them. In five categories, it suggests how many calories a week you need to burn through exercise, which could include running, to lower your risk factor of dying young and thus extending the length of your life.

Fitness category	Exercise calories	Equivalent in miles run	Risk factor	Extra years of life
Unfit	0	0	1.0	0
Somewhat fit	500	5	0.80	2
More fit	1,000	10	0.50	6
Still more fit	2,000	20	0.35	8
Superfit	3,500	35	0.25	9

his face. I had received a call from his office, saying my father had suffered a heart attack and had been rushed to the hospital. Three days later, he was dead.

By any measurement, Hig would have ranked as low fit, his chances of dying from a heart attack high. He never exercised. I have vague memories from when I was 2 or 3 years old seeing him at a playground near our apartment on the south side of Chicago playing in a softball game. He would have been around age 42, but beyond that my father's lifestyle was completely sedentary. He burned zero calories through exercise. During the last several decades of his life, he would come home from work on a Friday afternoon, get into his pajamas, and stay in them until Monday, when it was time to go to work again. Most of the time during the weekend, he puttered around the apartment, drinking beer: Carling's Red Cap Ale. He had a pot belly. He smoked most of his life. One day in his fifties he quit cold turkey, only to resume smoking again years later after my mother suffered a stroke, causing health problems that raised his stress level because he had to care for her.

Ironically, my mother outlived her husband by nearly a dozen years. She too was sedentary, her only physical activity participating in a weekly bowling league, hardly enough to generate the 2,000 exercise calories suggested by Dr. Paffenbarger. My mother's last years were not comfortable, her death supposedly from a heart attack at age 83 causing everybody at the wake to comment, "It's a blessing."

Yet I can hardly fault my parents; they were victims of their generation. They lived in an era that included the Roaring Twenties, a debilitating depression, and a world war. Scientists had not told them that by choosing a healthier lifestyle, they might have lived longer and better, and if they had been told, I'm not sure they would have paid much attention. Even today, too few people do. Among those who report to The Cooper Clinic for physical examinations and find their way into Dr. Blair's study, only 20 percent rank as moderately fit or high fit with accompanying longer life. Had my parents and I switched generations, I might never have become a runner or realized the benefits of exercise. I was the beneficiary of good luck—although this brings us back to A.J. Foyt's comment that luck is when preparation meets opportunity.

We all are victims and beneficiaries of our genetics, seemingly doomed to suffer the fates of our ancestors. I already have been diagnosed with coronary heart disease, the same as my mother and father. What I don't know is how soon it will kill me.

The average life expectancy of someone born in the United States is currently 77.4 years, according to S. Jay Olshansky, an epidemiologist at the University of Chicago. Men live to 74.7. Women live longer, to 79.9, according to current estimates. But that's on average, and those are estimates. I am cursed (or blessed) with my own genetics.

If we accept Dr. Paffenbarger's study of the Harvard alumni that suggests 2 to 3 extra years of life for those who exercise and add those years to the age my father died, that brings me to age 72, my age as I write these words. I've outlived at least one of my parents. But if we shift from pessimists to optimists and accept the suggestion that 9 to 10 years extra life is possible, I live to age 78 and beat by half a year Olshansky's estimate for men and women. Or consider the possibility that I inherited more of my mother's genes. That brings me close to age 90. Might I some day win a gold medal at the World Masters Championships in the M90 category? At that age, you often win medals simply by showing up.

In all honesty, winning another gold medal hardly motivates me any more. I'd like my wife and myself to live long enough to see our grandchildren graduated from college and happily married. So I run as many days as I comfortably can and fill in the spots between with other forms of exercise, including those morning walks to get the newspaper.

Dr. George Sheehan understood that longevity was only part of the answer to why we exercise. "Don't be concerned if running or exercise will add years to your life," he wrote in his book *Running and Being,* "Be concerned with adding life to your years." Dr. Sheehan also liked to quote William James, who said, "The strenuous life tastes better."

It certainly does.

4 COMPETITION

Masters Running Comes of Age through the Vision of a San Diego Attorney

I n the summer of 1972, I traveled to Europe with a team of masters athletes led by David H. R. Pain, the San Diego attorney who had several years before organized the first track-and-field meet for runners older than 40. Now Pain was spreading his message abroad: organizing a tour of American masters to compete in a series of track meets from England to Finland to Sweden to Denmark to Germany, planting in each country the seed of an idea that aging runners still could enjoy competition.

Ironically, the focus of Pain's tour originally had been the Olympic Games that same summer in Munich, Germany. An avid sports fan, Pain wanted to attend the Olympics and discovered that a number of his new friends, who had come to San Diego to compete, had the same desire. "I began planning a tour to Munich," Pain recalls. "Almost as an afterthought, I contacted several British veterans to see if they might stage a small track meet in London for our group en route." ("Veterans" was the term the British used to describe over-40 athletes, who until this point more often competed in road races rather than track-and-field meets.)

The Olympic tour proved so attractive that soon Pain had deposits from 200 travelers, so many that he couldn't obtain enough tickets to the track events in Munich to satisfy everybody. As an alternative, he began to explore other travel options, including additional masters competition in Finland, Sweden, and Denmark. The group would divide after the London meet, then reunite in Germany for several final races before heading home. That's when Pain discovered that most of his group preferred to compete in Scandinavia rather than go to Munich and watch younger athletes.

Because of work commitments, I joined the group only for the track meets in London, Helsinki, and Stockholm. My most telling memory came not on the track, but at London's Victoria Station, where we caught a train to the Crystal Palace Sports Centre. (The Crystal Palace previously had been the site of the 1908 Olympic Games.) While buying tickets, we stood in line dressed in our uniforms: red-white-and-blue sweat suits with "U.S. Masters" on the back, striped running shoes, tote bags for our spikes, some of us carrying javelins and poles.

Behind me in line, a woman asked her husband, "Who are all these people in the athletic uniforms?"

Her husband shrugged, "They can't be runners. They're too old."

That idea soon would fade. We were the first wave of a masters movement that eventually would engulf the world. That first masters meet of "world" stature in London attracted at best a few hundred competitors. Pain recalls 172 on his tour, including athletes from Canada, Australia, and New Zealand. He suspects that an equal number of British veterans competed, but only a handful from elsewhere in Europe. Today, most World Masters Championships attract nearly 6,000 competitors. Twelve thousand athletes participated in the 1993 meet in Miyazaki, Japan, although a majority were Japanese competing in a well-promoted marathon on the last day of the track competition.

CRAZY OLD COOTS

David H. R. Pain did not discover running for older athletes any more than Christopher Columbus discovered America. The Indians—and maybe a few Norwegians—were there before Columbus, and at least a few older athletes continued to compete in road races before Pain organized his first masters track meet. The Boston Marathon had its share of crazy old coots, who did not know when to quit.

> If you finished after Clarence DeMar at Boston, few people would be present to cheer you along the course.

In 1910, the sponsoring Boston Athletic Association even tried to ban Peter Foley, because at age 52, he was too old. Foley disguised himself by shaving his whiskers and ran anyway. The BAA eventually rescinded the ban.

The most famous masters marathoner of them all, of course, was Clarence DeMar, who won Boston seven times, lastly in 1930 at the age of 41. DeMar's winning time of 2:34:48 from that year would make most masters runners proud even today. DeMar continued to run Boston through most of his life, his final race coming in 1954 at the age of 65, when he placed 78th with a time of 3:58:34. Most of the nearly one million spectators who lined the course from Hopkinton to Boston each year during the DeMar era arrived in time to see the leaders, stayed long enough to cheer DeMar, then went home. If you finished after Clarence, few people would be present to cheer you along the course.

Equally remarkable was the record for longevity achieved by John A. Kelley at Boston. That's "Old John" A. Kelley to differentiate him from "Young John" J. Kelley, a competitor from my era who won Boston in 1957. Old John won Boston in 1935 and again in 1945. Three years after that, he made the U.S. Olympic team in the marathon, competing in the 1948 Games in London at the age of 40. Kelley placed in the top 10 at Boston 18 times, six of those top 10 finishes coming after the age of 40, one of them after 50. In 1962, when I placed 26th at Boston with a time of 2:45:21 at the age of 31, Old John finished 1 minute and one place in front of me at age 54. Was I embarrassed? I was proud to have finished that close.

None of us young studs considered it remarkable that Kelley was still able to beat us at such an advanced age. He was simply this friendly fellow who was happy to chat with us and offer training advice. I do admit that my eyebrows raised when a month later, he ran

2:37:42 to place fourth in the National AAU Marathon Championships in Yonkers, New York. With a seemingly endless string of hills in the closing miles beside the Hudson River, Yonkers ranks among the toughest courses I have run, particularly since the race usually was run midday in May, almost guaranteeing oppressively hot weather. Although not yet identified as a "masters" runner, Kelley did have our respect for his accomplishments regardless of age.

The record by Kelley that may never be matched is his having run Boston 61 times, the first in 1928 at the age of 20, when he failed to finish, the last in 1992 at the age of 84, when he ran 5:58:00. Somebody who, like Kelley, started young may some day run a 62nd Boston, but it is highly unlikely that the same individual also will have won the race twice. Kelley died in 2004 at the age of 97.

While the Boston Marathon and other road races in New England attracted an occasional over-40 runner, little or no competition existed for an older competitor in, say, the high jump or even the sprints. While stationed with the U.S. Army in Germany during the fall of 1955, I sometimes competed in *waldlauf*, cross-country races that usually had multiple events and distances, beginning with children, but also including a class for *altherren,* older men, those over the age of 45. Locked in my own world of elite competition, I paid the *altherren* little attention, considering their performances neither unique nor very remarkable. Like Kelley, they were just there, part of the racing scene. Because sports competition in Europe was centered around sports clubs rather than schools and universities, people of all ages felt free to participate in whatever competitions they could find. Indeed, when David Pain began to communicate in 1972 with German sportsmen to organize races for his traveling group, he had to talk hard to get them to divide races into 10-year age groups. The Germans were used to throwing runners of all ages into the same races.

After discharge in 1956, I returned home and began to compete for the University of Chicago Track Club.

> While the Boston Marathon attracted over-40 runners, little competition existed for older competitors in the high jump or the sprints.

One of my teammates and occasional training partners at the University's Stagg Field was Harry Price, a man in his forties, who had competed for Indiana University before World War II. Harry's main event was 440 yards, the linear equivalent of 400 meters. He had run 48.3 for 440 and 1:53.8 for the 440 and 880 while in college and still was hitting near those times as an over-40 runner. One year in a summer all-comer's track meet, we raced shoulder-to-shoulder in a 660-yard race. I forget who won, but that distance was the dividing line when we raced each other. With superior sprint speed, he ruled everything below 660; I ruled the distances above. Did it seem unusual that this old guy was out on the track with us each day in training? Like with Kelley in the Boston Marathon, we didn't give it much thought.

At age 43, Harry joined the Peace Corps and was sent to Nigeria to coach their track athletes. Although many of the fastest American black sprinters certainly have Nigerian blood, the nation had only begun to develop its athletes to where they could compete on the Olympic level. Harry trained with the Nigerian quarter-milers and had little trouble keeping up with them. Another Peace Corps volunteer said to Harry one day: "Either these guys are really bad, or you're really good."

No organized age-group competition existed at this time that would have permitted Harry to run against his age peers. He ran with us in open competition, often running a leg on a 4 × 440 relay team, taking his lumps as he did. Harry continued to compete as a quarter-miler in open track meets until age 50 and still exercises today, mostly walking, at age 83.

Unfortunately for Harry Price and others his age who might have enjoyed the sport of their youth, David H. R. Pain had not yet invented the masters movement.

ENTER DAVID PAIN

David H. R. Pain: When you encounter someone with two middle initials, you suspect he may have English connections. David Holland Rose Pain was born in Taplow, Buckinghamshire, England, on

July 31, 1922. When he was five, his family moved to Windsor, Ontario, where his father worked on a Ford assembly line. They later settled in California. (In *Fitness after Forty,* I devoted a chapter to David Pain and the 1972 European masters tour.)

Pain started his own gardening business while attending North Hollywood High School, prospering to the point where he had four assistants caring for 22 yards. His senior year, he quit attending classes though he stopped by daily for assignments. He would have graduated anyway had he not, early in 1941, enlisted in the U.S. Navy, which assigned him to the USS Mount Vernon, a luxury liner converted into a troop transport. On the day the Japanese attacked Pearl Harbor, Pain stood on the fantail of his ship off the South African coast and watched two torpedoes, fired by a lurking German submarine, narrowly miss blowing him to bits.

The Mount Vernon sailed into Singapore under fog that prevented attacking Japanese airplanes from locating them and deposited the last reinforcements to that city, men whose later prison experiences inspired *The Bridge on the River Kwai.* (One Australian soldier who fought at Singapore and spent 4 years as a Japanese prisoner of war was John Gilmour, a frequent gold medalist and record setter in world masters meets. Gilmour later wrote a book about his wartime experiences, *All in My Stride.*) Before Singapore fell, Pain's ship sailed to Port Said to pick up the famous "Rats of Tobruk," Australians who had spent 2 years defending that city against Rommel.

For 3 years, the Mount Vernon sailed the South Pacific, transporting fresh troops one direction, wounded the other, with David Pain more an observer than a participant in the shooting war. He finally applied for a commission through the Navy's V-12 program, attending college at Occidental and UCLA. Ninety days before earning his commission, he became eligible for discharge. Having previously dropped out of high school, he now dropped out of college, but nevertheless earned entry to the University of Southern California Law School, where he met his future wife, Helen. He married Helen the following spring, honeymooned one weekend in San Diego, and after graduation (his first) began practicing law in that city.

While establishing his own law firm in Ocean Beach, Pain supplemented the family diet, and satisfied his own competitive urge, by surfing and spearfishing. His law practice gradually expanded, and he added several partners, including Bob Pippin, who climbed mountains in his spare time. "He's a good lawyer in the courtroom," claimed Pippin. "He's tenacious at digging out details." Pain was tenacious enough to have been threatened more than once for contempt of court. On one occasion, Pain helped win the largest wrongful-death verdict in San Diego County: $470,000 to the widow of a man killed in a commercial airline crash.

Frequent colds caused Pain to abandon water sports. He learned to fly. As a Los Angeles Rams season ticket-holder, he often went to games by air. On one occasion, Pain found himself lost above the overcast in his Beechcraft Bonanza with a failing battery, a non-functioning radio, and his entire family. Fortunately, a hole appeared in the clouds, enabling him to land in El Cajon just east of San Diego. The experience sobered him. He sold the plane, a decision made easier by the arrival in town of the San Diego Chargers.

Pain began playing handball and soon was serving as club handball commissioner, organizing competitive trips to Los Angeles and San Francisco. But soon he tired of that sport. "First, I wasn't getting enough exercise. Second, it was too much of a hassle reserving courts and locating opponents. Third, I was getting home too late evenings. I started jogging mornings with my dog."

It did not take David Pain long to locate other joggers. One of them was Augie Escamilla, a student counselor at San Diego State, who worked out Sunday mornings with a group of older runners. Pain reflects wistfully: "There was something about being able to run on a beach or in a park in the quiet of nature that totally relieves you of the burdens of modern living. You develop an inner peace. You eliminate the turmoil and emotional stress."

Running also caused Pain to abandon his seat on the 50-yard line at Charger games. "I'd decided to become a participant rather than an observer," he says. Jogging, however, failed to satisfy Pain's natural competitive urge the way handball did. Handball players were much better organized competitively. They even had special categories for players over 40. The handball players used the term "masters" to describe players in that category.

The U.S. Handball Association added a masters category to its national championships in 1952 in recognition of the fact that handball, because of the many bounces a ball can take off four surrounding walls, was a very difficult game to master. Once a player learns the angles, however, he often can play a control-pattern game,

MASTERS MILES

Twenty thousand spectators watched the first masters mile orchestrated by David H. R. Pain in 1966 as part of a popular San Diego track-and-field meet that attracted some of the fastest runners in the world. Les Land was meet director. Pain recalls: "I approached Land with the idea of adding a race for runners over 40. He was lukewarm until I suggested the name 'masters mile.' That hooked him. Although we played second fiddle to the likes of Peter Snell, Jim Ryun, Billy Mills, and Gerry Lindgren, the catchy name found its way into wire-service reports. As a result, open track meets elsewhere began including the event, spurring interest in masters athletics."

One individual contacting Pain for suggestions the following year was Jim Hartshorne, an ornithologist from Ithaca, New York, home of Cornell University. Hartshorne talked the track coach at Cornell into inserting a masters mile into a major indoor meet limited to college athletes.

"The race proved successful," wrote Rick Hoebeke in the newsletter of the Finger Lakes Runners, "so Jim got on the telephone to race directors of all the major track meets on the East Coast in an attempt to sell them the idea."

Not all race directors were impressed. "I don't want some old fart dropping dead on my track," said one. But within a few years several major meets added masters events, including the Knights of Columbus Games in Boston, the Millrose Games in New York, and the Penn Relays in Philadelphia.

I met Jim Hartshorne during David Pain's European tour. He talked me

rarely having to move more than a step or two in either direction. Shrewd, mature players thus can play handball against faster, yet less-experienced, players without excessive strain. Masters competition proved so popular that the USHA later added golden masters (50 and over) and super masters (60 and over) divisions at its national championships.

David Pain reasoned logically: If such age divisions worked for

into coming to his masters mile, which conveniently was after another masters mile in an indoor track meet in Philadelphia that I ran several times. In my first Philadelphia appearance, Jim Hershberger of Kansas and I ran a near dead heat, both lunging for the tape, falling and skidding across the boards. These were old men? The crowd loved it.

Even better was the same masters mile in Philadelphia 2 years later. I held the lead into the last lap when Henry Kupczyk, a Polish Olympian emigrated to the United States, passed on the outside of the final turn and shoved me into the infield. Moving back on the track, I pushed Henry, unfortunately propelling him forward, so he beat me. Despite finishing one-two, we were disqualified, the win going to Frank Pflagling, who also had won the previous year. I argued with officials that Henry had been disqualified at the time of the first push, so I too shouldn't have been disqualified, since technically he was no longer in the race when I fouled him. Somehow, they failed to appreciate the logic of my argument.

After the Philadelphia race in 1973, I traveled to Ithaca to run at Cornell, placing second to Hal Snyder. Jim Hartshorne had competed in the first masters track-and-field meet in San Diego in 1968, winning the mile in 4:50.5. He was a single father charged with raising three young children, his wife having died in an accident. The Cornell Masters Mile continued under Hartshorne's direction, and in 1981 he added a women's mile that attracted nine competitors. Rick Hoebeke of the Finger Lakes Runners took over management of the races in 1991, which became the Hartshorne Memorial Masters Miles after Jim's death 3 years later. The race continues to this day, the oldest men's as well as women's masters miles in North America, perhaps in the world.

handball, why wouldn't they be appropriate for track and field? He approached Les Land, promoter of the San Diego outdoor meet, with this radical idea in 1966. Land agreed to add a mile run for older runners.

It was an idea whose time had come. The masters mile was reasonably popular with spectators, but even more so with competitors. Masters miles soon sprung up in other parts of the country. Jim Hartshorne, who would become a participant on Pain's 1972 European tour, organized a masters mile at an indoor track meet at Cornell University in Ithaca, New York, starting in January 1968. But it was David Pain who later that summer of 1968 took one step further and organized a full-event masters track-and-field meet.

A SMATTERING OF OLYMPIANS

Competition at this first championship for older runners was spotty and sometimes amusing. Not all the masters took themselves seriously. One runner appeared for the start of the 100-yard dash wearing house slippers with elastic bands to keep them on his feet. A shot putter sewed lace on his gym shorts. A smattering of Olympians—George Rhoden, Bob Richards, Bud Held—added class to early meets, but most participants had not competed in 20 years, and others never had tried the sport.

One of my former training partners from the U.C.T.C. ran the 3-mile and 6-mile in that first masters meet. Harold Harris, several years older than I, had competed for the University of Illinois and continued in track meets and road races after graduation. Harold was a good journeyman runner, whose peak moment of glory came at the 1964 Olympic marathon trials in Yonkers, New York. Buddy Edelen, world record holder at the time, pushed the pace on a day where the temperature hit 95, luring many of the faster runners out with him. I ran with Buddy through the first 10 miles, but the heat soon got to me. Still in second place at 17 miles, my ears started to ring. I slowed down, and the ringing stopped. I sped up, and the ringing started again. This happened several times before I finally pulled off the course. Norman Higgins went by me and held second place for several miles before the course turned left, and he continued to run straight—into a wall. Norm reportedly was in a hospital for a week.

> The masters mile was reasonably popular with spectators, but even more so with competitors.

Harold Harris, however, started slowly and after a few miles was running around 50th place, as officials along the way told him. As the race continued, he moved into 25th place, then the top 10. "I couldn't understand it," Harold told me afterward, "because I wasn't passing anybody!" Of the 128 who started the race, only 37 finished. Harold finished fourth with a time of 2:55. Edelen won in 2:24:26, a remarkable time given the conditions, earning a spot on the U.S. Olympic team that competed in Tokyo later that summer. (A separate Olympic trial in California contributed two other marathoners to the team.) Edelen never fully recovered from that effort. One of the favorites for the gold medal because of his world record the previous year, he struggled home sixth in Tokyo.

Four years later at the first masters track-and-field meet in San Diego, Harold Harris placed second in both the 3-mile and 6-mile behind Peter Mundle. Another runner who traveled to San Diego in 1968 was John A. Kelley, then 60. Old John ran 3:04:33 to place third overall in the marathon behind Richard Packard and Alex Ratelle. Seventh overall in that same race was Bill Andberg, 57, new to running, although he had participated in snowshoe races as a youngster. Andberg, of Anoka, Minnesota, would come to dominate his age groups in the next several decades, winning four World Masters Championships and setting 22 American records at distances from 800 meters through the 30-K. (Andberg was among the athletes recruited by Mike Pollock for his study of aging.)

As the masters movement progressed, competition became tougher. New athletes appeared who would not sew lace on their shorts. Thane Baker, a silver medalist in the 200 meters at the 1952 and 1956 Olympic Games and a 4 × 100 relay gold medalist, appeared on the scene to dominate the sprints. (Baker also was one of the athletes being tested in the Mike Pollock study.) Yet while improving in excellence, the masters movement did not lose its humanity: Joggers still remained much a part of the scene. The masters movement also created an anomaly: men in their late 30s eagerly anticipating their 40th birthday.

By 1971, David Pain obtained the blessing of the Amateur Athletic Union to recognize his meet as a true national championships. He also succeeded in convincing the AAU to amend its rules to permit professionals (assuming they were over 40) to compete in masters competition. Former professional boxer Chuck Davey, who once fought Kid Gavilan for the world middleweight title, began to compete as a masters runner. Miler Wes Santee, barred by the AAU in the mid-1950s for accepting money, returned to competition, running masters miles on several occasions at the Kansas Relays. Many track coaches, at one time also considered "professionals," found they could run again. Among them was Stanford and Olympic coach Payton Jordan, a world record-holder in his youth. Jordan soon began setting world records for 50-year-old sprinters and continued doing so through his 60s and 70s.

Another Stanford graduate and sprinter who competed in masters track at that time was Alan Cranston, a member of the U.S. Senate. Senator Cranston is best remembered for appearing in a 50-meter dash for athletes over 50 at an indoor track meet in San Francisco. Pulling down his sweat pants before taking his place in the blocks, Cranston inadvertently yanked his shorts down, mooning nearly 10,000 spectators. It didn't seem to hurt him in his election campaign.

Though considered by many to be the father of the masters movement, David Pain did not claim all the credit when I interviewed him for a *Runner's World* article back in the 1970s. "It's not enough just to have a good idea," he said. "It has to come along at the right time. But I do think masters track is the most significant new thing to arise in a very old sport. People now can continue to participate even though their abilities have diminished. And this is the secret of masters track, something that we must never lose sight of. It's the secret of age-group competition. We have had age-group competition for years with kids. Now we have all these old guys competing and having a wonderful time, because now they can win an event instead of being at the back of the pack.

"It's a chance to relive their youth. Either they missed athletics as a youth, like me, or they were in athletics and enjoyed it, and this provides a chance to get back. There is a certain camaraderie in the sport, which is what gives me the motivation to try and stay fit. I don't think I'd train as hard if it were not for some upcoming races. I probably wouldn't travel. I'd stay home or go backpacking somewhere on holiday. Now, I've become a world traveler as a result of the masters movement."

WORLD TRAVELERS

For the 1972 masters tour to Europe, Helen and David Pain secured a charter flight. We shared the plane with a group of Stanford alumni. Smoking still was allowed on airplanes back then, and Pain almost came to blows with some of the alumni smoking cigarettes.

I chatted with Thane Baker, who had retired soon after the 1956 Olympics, returning to competition only after turning 40. Much had changed during Thane's retirement, including tracks: dirt and cinder during his Olympic years, now constructed of various synthetic compounds that provided a firmer, yet bouncier surface. The long, ⅝-inch spikes used decades before had been replaced with shorter ¼-inch spikes. "I've never run on an all-weather track before," Thane confessed to me halfway across the Atlantic. "I don't even own a pair of shoes with short spikes yet." When we landed in London, one of his first priorities would be finding a sporting goods store.

Also on the flight was Roland Anspach, who then worked for General Motors in Dayton, Ohio. When he turned 40, Roland began to run, even though he never had competed in track before. "It was something I always had wanted to do," he told me. "At first, I trained while delivering my son's paper route so the neighbors wouldn't think me crazy."

After 6 months' preparation, Roland entered his first race, a masters mile at Ohio University. He ran 5:50. Four years later, he ran on a 24-hour relay team, averaging 5:27 for 25 separate miles. He no longer delivered newspapers, saying: "The neighbors are used to me now."

Jim O'Neil of Sacramento, California, had attended the University of Miami, where he was number three runner on a cross-country team that ran only one meet a season. He claimed to be running faster at age 47 than he had in college. (A participant in the first national championships in 1971, O'Neil has run every national meet since then through 2004, as well as every world meet.)

"There always have been opportunities for older distance runners," Jim commented to me, "but the good thing about the masters program is it gives the sprinters and jumpers a chance to compete again."

BORN OF FRUSTRATION

My motivation to compete past the age of 40 was born partly out of frustration from having been an underachiever in my twenties and thirties. I had started my running career late, not having taken the sport too seriously in high school when I failed to break 5:00 for the mile. I ran 5:04.3 as a sophomore, but skipped track my junior year and failed to improve as a senior. While attending a small college, I sliced more than a half-minute off that time, good enough to win races against other small-college athletes, but not against national class performers. World class? I barely knew what the term meant.

Continuing to run after graduation, I achieved some success but seemed always a step or two behind the top performers. My breakthrough nationally was fifth in the 10,000 at the AAU Championships in 1954. I placed fifth in the 3000-meter steeplechase at the 1960 Olympic trials, but only three made the team. I placed fifth in the 1964 Boston Marathon after leading through 19 miles, but failed to achieve my goal of winning it. Definitely, I was a fifth-rate runner. In two Olympic years I had times faster than those of runners who made the

"At first, I trained while delivering my son's paper route so the neighbors wouldn't think me crazy."

American team, but I failed in the trials. Injuries seemed to plague me at the wrong time. My failures, I deduced later, were partly because of overtraining. My Protestant work ethic was too strong—and I wasn't even Protestant! By the time I figured out how to train properly, I was in my mid-thirties, and younger runners began to eclipse me. When I turned 40, I grasped at masters running as a way to redeem myself for failed opportunities.

Many of us who traveled to Europe with David Pain during the summer of 1972 had similar stories. After a cross-country race and 2-day track meet at the Crystal Palace in London, we flew to Helsinki for another track meet, then took a boat to Stockholm. The Olympic Games had begun in Munich, and for a while we were close enough to shore to watch the competition being broadcast by a Finnish TV station. But the picture soon faded, and I found myself talking with Alphonse Juilland, then head of Stanford's linguistics department.

As a boy, Alphonse competed in the sprints in his native France, but World War II halted a promising athletic career. He began jogging again at Stanford, got to know members of the track team, and one day attended the West Coast Relays to watch decathlete Bill Toomey perform.

The program featured a 100-yard dash for senior runners, and several of Alphonse's students pulled him out of the stands, demanding he compete. Wearing a borrowed pair of shoes, he placed second, pulling a leg muscle while doing so. But the competitive bug had struck. Alphonse set his goal at running 11.0 for 100 yards, and while 50 years old he ran that distance in 10.5 seconds. (One hundred yards is approximately 10 yards shorter than the now more frequently run 100 meters. Juilland's 100-yard time of 10.5 would convert to about 11.5 for the slightly longer distance.)

Considering Alphonse's muscle pull, I questioned him about the dangers that older athletes faced by taking part in an explosive event like the 100-yard dash. Long-distance runners, at least a few of us, had continued to run races as we aged. Only recently had sprinters like Alphonse been lured back into competition. Nobody in his right mind, I suggested, would attempt a marathon without training for it.

But someone with more fast-twitch muscles, and also perhaps more testosterone, might be lured out of the stands into a sprint event under the perhaps flawed assumption that anyone could run 100 yards, even without training. Are we kidding ourselves in motivating grandfather jocks to do something that was better left undone?

"I'll admit some danger," Alphonse smiled. "But older sprinters must prepare for competition by becoming long-distance runners first—then working down to shorter distances at faster speeds. They probably should obtain a thorough medical checkup before starting—not just a regular electrocardiogram, but a dynamic electrocardiogram in which a trained physiologist monitors the heart under exercise."

Alphonse continued to say that we harbor too many fears about what men older than 40 could accomplish. "We age ourselves prematurely by thinking old," he lectured, citing the example of Adolfo Consolini, who at age 47 still held the Italian record in the discus and continued to throw. "He was the best thrower in his country and

CREATIVE COMPETITION

American masters who got their first exposure to international competition after crossing the Atlantic Ocean often were surprised to discover that Europeans seemed to operate under different rule books. Approaching a street corner in a masters 25-K race in Bruges, Belgium, I watched as a continental runner cut across a sidewalk and lawn. British runners near me were outraged, but there was little we could do.

Having competed on the European track circuit while younger, I knew distance running often was a contact sport. One notorious photo taken a fraction of a second after the start of the M40 cross-country race at the 1977 World Masters Championships in Gothenburg, Sweden, shows competitors grasping and clawing at each other as though in a rugby scrum.

I ran the M45 race that same day and reacted slowly to the gun, finding myself behind several dozen runners when we funneled into a tight trail. Blocked, I could do little more than coast helplessly as the leaders sprinted away on the two-lap, 10,000-meter course.

one of the best in the world," Alphonse commented. "But according to Italy's athletic rules, nobody past the age of 45 could compete, so Adolfo had to join a Swiss club and compete in his home country as a foreigner."

We docked in Stockholm and, after a track meet in the Olympic stadium used for the 1912 Games where I got outkicked in the 1500 meters, I flew home. Pain and his merry men continued on to Denmark and Germany. We had begun to change attitudes at least among countries in Western Europe as to what older athletes could and couldn't do. Although pockets of competition for masters (or veteran) runners already existed throughout Europe and in other parts of the world, the 1972 tour would set in motion events that would result, within 3 years, in a fully international masters movement.

A key meeting occurred while we were in London during the time period between a cross-country race in Epping Forest and the 2-day track meet at the Crystal Palace. Playing Boswell to David Pain's Samuel Johnson, I was invited to join a group meeting at a local pub.

It took me the entire first lap to move into what was fourth place, except the top three runners remained out of sight on the course that wound through woods and meadow. Hard as I ran, I couldn't catch them, see them, nor, strangely, could I gain much on those behind. Our course was defined by flags delineating turns that forced us to zigzag back and forth. I ran around each flag, but looking over my shoulder, I realized nobody else possessed the same scruples. Did this include the leaders? I don't know, but I finished fourth, missing a medal by one place.

Four years later at the Worlds in Christchurch, New Zealand, Roger Robinson of the host country used an interesting tactic while winning M40 cross-country. To add a degree of difficulty to a flat course, meet organizers included three steeplechase barriers. I didn't run cross-country, but watched as Roger ducked under the barriers rather than hurdling them. "I checked the rules," Roger told me afterward. "They say you have to 'negotiate' the barriers. They didn't say how." Since Roger probably used more energy going under rather than over, I hardly can accuse him of winning unfairly.

In addition to Pain, the group included Donald Farquharson, head of the Canadian team, and Wal Sheppard, head of the Australian team. Hosting the meeting were Jack Fitzgerald and Jack Hayward of the British veterans organization. Unique about this group was the fact that not only were these team leaders organizing the track meet, they all were running in it! (Baron Pierre de Coubertin failed to run in the Olympic Games he promoted in Athens, Greece in 1896.)

As our group sipped pints of British ale, we talked first about plans for the track meet scheduled within a few days: seeding athletes into heats, discussing eligibility. Accompanying us on the trip was Bill Gookin, a distance runner from San Diego who was several weeks short of his 40th birthday. (Bill, a chemist, later would achieve a certain sense of fame by developing a sports replacement drink, popular among runners, called E.R.G. for Electrolyte Replacement with Glucose, also known as Gookinaid.) Ever persuasive, Pain coaxed the usually more stringent Brit vets into allowing Gookin to compete unofficially.

Then as the pints of ale continued to appear on the table, we began to consider the future of masters track and field. Pain's vision extended beyond 1972. That weekend's track meet was, at best, an unofficial "world" masters championships, as had his 1968 meet in San Diego been an unofficial "national" championships. We discussed organizing a true World Masters Championships, open to all athletes over the age of 40. Before the pints were dry, it had been decided to hold such an event. Donald Farquharson promised that he would return to Toronto to begin planning an international track meet, which became a reality in 1975. Two years later at the second championships in Sweden, Farquharson would be elected as president of the newly formed World Association of Veteran Athletes (WAVA), a position he held for 10 years.

The organization adopted the British term "veteran," rather than the American term "masters," to describe those eligible to participate: men over 40 and women over 35. No women had participated in the Crystal Palace meet, and few would appear in 1975 in Toronto. To encourage women, they were permitted to enter at an earlier age. "Some of the older men had younger wives or girlfriends," Pain explained. Eventually, the name of the organization would be changed to World Masters Association and the age at which people could

> Are we kidding ourselves in motivating grandfather jocks to do something that was better left undone?

compete equalized at 35 for men and women.

But that was far in the future. During the 1972 tour to Europe, I continued to exorcise the demons that had plagued me as a younger runner. No more fifth places, I vowed. Skipping the cross-country race at Epping Forest on Tuesday, I focused on the 3000-meter steeplechase Friday and won comfortably over Australia's Ron Young. My time of 9:36.2 set a world M40 record, less impressive when you consider that few runners over 40 had run that event in competition before. (Five years later in Sweden, Gaston Roelants of Belgium would run a much more respectable 8:45, still the M40 world record.) Saturday, I finished fourth (not fifth) in the 5000 meters behind three British athletes, but my time of 14:59.6 would remain an American M40 record for nearly a quarter-century.

WE WERE MASTERS

I still had a few more demons circling my shoulder as we arrived in Helsinki for a track meet at the 1952 Olympic stadium. I had competed in Finland with an American team in 1956, winning three of five races, but none of those races was in the Olympic stadium. I might not have been good enough to compete on that hallowed track while younger, but I could do so as a masters runner.

Among those running against me in a 10,000 were Bill Allen of Canada, Bill Gookin, the almost-40 San Diegoan, and a runner wearing the traditional white Finnish uniform with light blue cross on the singlet. This was enough to bring fear to the heart of any distance runner. In the first half of the 20th century, despite the small size of their country, Finns had dominated distance running on the track with runners like Kolehmainen, Ritola, Nurmi. They were like the Kenyans today. They also dominated the Boston Marathon, two

Finns having finished in front of me in 1964 when I placed fifth.

But this was 1972, and we were masters. The starter motioned for us to position ourselves on the white line drawn across the rust-colored track. We wished each other good luck, then the gun sounded. Is it possible to conjure exact details of a race that happened more than 3 decades ago? My training diary offers little help. It was night, but it couldn't have been dark, because the sun hardly sets at Helsinki's northern latitude in the summer. The huge stadium was near empty, because who wants to watch a bunch of runners over 40? That lap times were announced in Finnish didn't matter. As we circled lap after inexorable lap, 25 of them, I could see the scoreboard clock as we passed the start-finish line. We rolled around the track at a steady 5:00 per mile pace, faster than my best times from high school. What tactical moves did I make? Most likely I followed the pace of the other runners, yet occasionally moved to the front to "take a pull," as the Brits like to say.

But on that evening, I had the best kick and moved past Allen, then the Finnish runner in the last lap, cruising to victory. My time of 31:18.4 was another American record.

But records are for statisticians, not athletes. My fast time was secondary to the fact that I had triumphed in the Olympic stadium over a good masters field, if not the world's best who were running against each other at the same time in Munich. The Finnish runner came over to congratulate me. He spoke no English; I spoke no Finnish. I came to realize that his name was Paavo Pystynen. He pointed his finger at me, then himself, and said the word, "Boston."

Then I remembered another day at Boston 8 years before, my fastest marathon, but also one of my many failures. I led at 19 miles and up the second Newton hill, only to be passed by the defending champion and eventual winner: Aurele Vandendriessche of Belgium. Then a Finnish runner passed, then a Canadian runner, then a second Finnish runner as I sank to fifth place, defeated in my bid for victory. An

> We are all champions. We are never defeated, no matter how many of our competitors finish in front of us.

Argentinean runner was about to catch me. Behind him was Young John Kelley. I was toast. Cresting Heartbreak Hill at 21 miles, I easily could have dropped out. I had done so on my first two runs at Boston. But I recovered, both physically and mentally, and in the last few miles coming down Commonwealth Avenue, I set my eyes on the second Finnish runner, hoping to catch him and improve my position.

I never did. That second runner was Paavo Pystynen.

Thus I had waited 8 years and come halfway around the world to finally catch that runner, exorcising at least one more demon. But it's unfair to speak of a fellow masters runner as a demon. I didn't feel that I had defeated Paavo Pystynen that evening in Helsinki. Nor did I feel I had defeated any of the other athletes whom I might have raced as a young runner and whom I would continue to race as an older runner, even until this day.

We are all champions. We are never defeated, no matter how many of our competitors finish in front of us. Vince Lombardi reportedly once said "winning is the only thing," but as a football coach, how would he know what motivates masters runners? I'm not even sure what motivates me any more, unless it is love, a zest for life, a desire to do as best as I can on every day of my life remaining. For this, I have David H. R. Pain to thank.

5 TRAINING

It Sometimes Takes a Lifetime to Learn How to Train Properly

My introduction to training theory began on the infield grass of the University of California, Berkeley. The year was 1952. I was a junior at Carleton College, a small college in Northfield, Minnesota with only 850 students. I was in Berkeley to participate in the NCAA Track and Field Championships. Carleton competed in the Midwest Conference against schools its own size. Only a few weeks before, I had won conference titles in the mile and 880, but this was the big time. In Berkeley, I would be running against much faster runners: athletes on scholarship from schools such as Southern California, Kansas, Michigan, Villanova, Georgetown, and Yale.

I was not so much badly beaten as I was seriously outclassed. Not only were most of the scholarship athletes who finished in front of me more talented, but they were better coached, better trained, and certainly more dedicated to their craft than I, a part-time runner. In one event, the 5000 meters, I actually finished in last place! Years later, I wrote an article on the experience for *Sports Illustrated,* and titled it "A Time of Wonder, Joy, and Glory for Losers."

But I learned lessons that later I would use as a masters runner. Not willing to believe that the scholarship athletes were that much more talented, I sat on the infield grass and quizzed them about the training that had brought them to such heights. My coaches at Carleton—Cy DeCoster in cross-country and Wally Hass in track—were reasonably knowledgeable individuals, but they were dealing with student-athletes who, like me, had "wandered" out for the team, whose goals were more academic than athletic. Well-intentioned all of us, but you're not going to win an NCAA championship or make an Olympic team if that is your main focus.

Among those athletes I engaged in conversation while seated on the infield grass was Frank McBride, a distance runner from South Dakota State. I had raced against Frank frequently in the upper Midwest, but never had beaten him. A 4:14 miler, he would place sixth in the 1500 meters at the Olympic trials a few weeks later. Through Frank, I got to know friends of his from San Diego State and through them, other athletes at major universities. Most of the conversations about training were brief and have faded from my memory, but one important fact sticks out even to this day. It is a fact so obvious that if you mentioned it to even the slowest jogger or the newest marathon wannabe, he would wonder why an athlete from a college with such high academic standards as Carleton had not figured it out on his own.

The athletes beating me all trained year-round. If they didn't run 12 months of the year, they certainly ran 11. Their breaks, if any, rarely lasted more than a week or two at a time, the breaks mainly to refresh themselves mentally so they could train harder for their next goal.

In contrast, I was a part-time runner, a parvenu, running at most 6 to 8 months a year, training maybe 15 to 20 miles a week maximum. Rest is good, but my approach might better be identified as abandonment. I would appear for cross-country practice in the fall, not having run a step the entire summer. My teammates, I'm sure, did the same. Once that season ended in early November, I would stop running, not to start again until the beginning of the indoor track season in January.

Each year at semester break, nearly 25 percent of the college piled on buses for a week of skiing at Mount Telemark in Cable, Wisconsin. My reaction was: Sign me up! Did it occur to me that a bad fall might end the track season for the year? Certainly not, plus at that age, who cares? On one of the ski trips I con-nected with the gal who

> The athletes beating me all trained year-round. Their breaks, if any, rarely lasted more than a week or two.

became my steady date the rest of the school year. A man must have priorities, and running was not at the top of my list most of my college career.

After outdoor track ended in May, I would quit again until it was time to return to school in September. Why run when it interfered with my other after-work summer activities such as golf, tennis, and hanging out at the beach with the girls?

Returning home from California, I still did not run much that summer, but in my senior year, my priorities began to shift. During the cross-country season, I started to add long runs on Sundays, dragging a few of my teammates along for the ride. By any standard our runs were not "long," probably a half-dozen miles maximum, less than an hour's worth of running, but this was more than any of us had done before. Once the cross-country season ended, I continued to run, bridging the gap between that sport and the track season. If that doesn't sound like much of a commitment, you have never run through a Minnesota winter!

My times did not improve significantly my senior year, but my performances certainly did. I rarely got beat, doubling in most dual meets to score team points. I achieved a level of consistency in my training and my racing. At the Midwest Conference Championships that spring, I repeated as mile champion and finished one-two in the 2-mile with teammate Ben Nelson, who also had benefited from those winter workouts. We were trying to tie for first, but the officials awarded the title to Ben, which was okay with me, because Carleton won the team title, its first in 18 years.

Examine that paragraph above and you will spot a word that was most important to my success and that of my teammates, but which is even more important to those of you who aspire to success as masters runners. That word is: consistency!

STARTING TO TRAIN

Although I ran two seasons of track in high school, my life as a runner didn't seriously begin until I arrived at Carleton College in the fall of 1949. It seems ridiculous now, but I actually debated whether to go out for football or cross-country. Thus, I joined the cross-country team several days late. By the end of the week, however, I had established myself as the fastest runner on the freshman squad.

My coach was Cy DeCoster, a gentle man, whose main duty was teaching languages. Because he had run in college, the athletic department recruited him as an unpaid volunteer to coach cross-country. Also helping with the freshmen was Bill "Pinky" Hendren, the fastest runner on the varsity team.

One of my teammates and later roommates was Lou McMurray, who still participates in road races and triathlons. At our 50th class reunion, we ran a 5-K race together. After the reunion, Lou bicycled from Northfield, Minnesota, back home to Peoria, Illinois, a distance of 520 miles, which he covered in 9 days.

Lou remembers our training at Carleton: "We went long at the start of the week, then tapered toward the weekend's race." We ran most of our workouts on trails through the Cowling Arboretum, circling Lyman Lakes, a

A LEVEL OF CONSISTENCY

If you fail to achieve consistency in your training, you are doomed to a lower level of achievement—as I had discovered when I competed in the 1952 NCAA Championships. A catchphrase in the new millennium is 24/7: 24 hours a day, 7 days a week. Obviously you can't devote anywhere near that amount of time to training, but you do need that same level of commitment. This is the first secret of masters success: You need to train year-round. Masters runners particularly don't need to train every day, since occasional and well-planned days off can contribute to fitness, but they need to train most days. Vitally important, they need to avoid long periods when they fail to run, or at least participate in some form of cross-training.

bucolic setting that I appreciate more and more the longer I am away from it. The freshmen raced on a 2-mile course; the varsity raced 3 miles, adding the extra distance with two loops around the athletic field. I recall our workouts in somewhat more detail than Lou.

Monday—Overdistance: 4 miles, or two laps around the Arb

Tuesday—Underdistance: 2 miles, or one lap at a faster pace

Wednesday—Mid-distance: 3 miles, the varsity course

Thursday—Repeats: 2 × ¾ mile, the athletic field loop

Friday—Rest: to get ready for Saturday's race

Saturday—Competition: Race 3 miles

Sunday—Rest: to recover from Saturday's race

Given the fact that we probably jogged a mile or so to warm up and maybe a half-mile to cool down, the team ran 15–20 miles a week. That's not a bad starting program for a beginning runner, whether student, adult, or master. It helped me win a Midwest Conference cross-country championship my senior year.

Scientific research suggests that after a period of detraining, you need to retrain 2 days for every 1 day you lost to regain previous fitness.

That was one of the main factors that limited my success as a college athlete. The lack of consistency in my training meant I was constantly starting over at the beginning of each season. I would retain some conditioning from the previous season, but not enough to allow me to progress to the limits of my ability. A chart of my annual progress was like a jagged line angled somewhat upward, permitting some improvement, but not like an ever upward moving stairway that would have allowed me to reach the top sooner.

The training lesson I learned on the infield grass at Berkeley is even more important to masters runners, those of us trying to maintain our competitive edge for as many years as possible. Research cited earlier in this book suggests that we achieve our peak performances between the ages of 20 and 40. After that, it is a matter of trying to stay as close to that peak as possible. The few times as a master I took a month or two off because of injury or because I needed a rest from hard training, I was unable to regain my previous peak. The jagged line had tilted downward. Accepting such a drop was largely my own choice, dictated by other priorities, yet if you want to achieve success as a masters runner, you don't necessarily have to train hard, but you need to be consistent about your training.

Had I abandoned my career as a competitive athlete after graduating from college—as most runners did in that era—my knowledge of what constituted proper training would have ended at that point. You would not be reading this book, because I would not have been smart enough to write it. But by the time of my graduation from Carleton in 1953, I started to realize that I had only begun to tap my athletic potential, that I might reach greater heights if new competitive opportunities presented themselves.

Alas, unlike today, few such opportunities presented themselves for track athletes or distance runners back in the 1950s unless you were Olympic caliber, good enough to have your expenses paid to major track meets: indoor meets, largely on the East Coast, or outdoor meets, largely on the West Coast. Road runners also had few opportunities in that era unless they lived in or near New England, the only area of the United States where (partly because of the long shadow cast by the Boston Marathon) a well-organized road-racing circuit served their needs. Not only was I not good enough yet to gain entry to the major track meets, I didn't live in New England.

A LIBERAL APPROACH TO ATHLETICS

Fortunately, I did have one option. The University of Chicago under the leadership of Chancellor Robert Maynard Hutchins marched to a different drumbeat from that of most educational institutions. You could skip grades and enter the university at a young age if you could pass their entrance exams. I had spent 2 years (9th and 10th grades) at the university's Laboratory School (U-High), but transferred to another high school rather than enter college 2 years early. Students at the U. of C. under the Hutchins regimen progressed from degree to degree to degree by testing out of classes. If they were smart enough, they could earn a college degree in a year. My high-school girlfriend, a former Quiz Kid, was 2 years younger than I but graduated from college 2 years before me.

Matching this liberal approach to education was a liberal approach to athletics. The glory days of Amos Alonzo Stagg on the gridiron had passed, but if you wanted to compete as an athlete at the University of Chicago, the school offered 4 years of eligibility whether or not you were an undergraduate or in graduate school. Again, it was Hutchins thumbing his nose at the educational establishment. NCAA rules at that time permitted only 3 years' eligibility, freshmen not being allowed to compete. As a result, many track athletes looking to extend their competitive years flocked to graduate programs at Chicago. I chose that route, and so did the runner who had won the 10,000 meters at the 1952 NCAA Championships: Walt Deike. Walt enrolled in medical school, but continued to run track and cross-country. Also training at Stagg Field in the fall of 1953 was Lawton Lamb, who had run on a record-setting 4 × 880 relay team for the University of Illinois. Lawton was trying to make his mark as a miler on the indoor track circuit. Jim Flynn was the top varsity cross-country runner at Chicago until I arrived, and we trained frequently together. It was because of the opportunity to train daily with better runners that I took the next step upward. They pulled me to faster times.

Consider that the second secret of achieving success as a masters runner: Work out with better training partners. Or at least, train with the best ones you can find. It doesn't matter whether they are younger or older than you, somewhat slower or somewhat faster, even of the same sex. You can push yourself harder in workouts with someone by your side near your equal in ability. It's

> Masters runners don't need to train every day, but they need to train most days.

worth the time and effort to climb in a car to meet with such training partners, even if only 1 day a week.

During this first year in graduate school, I came under the influence of E. Morgan Haydon, the varsity coach at the University of Chicago. "Ted" Haydon had run track and played football under Amos Alonzo Stagg in the 1930s, while majoring in sociology. More for fun than from any serious Olympic aspirations, and long before there was any masters competition, Ted used to throw the hammer. It was also a good way for him to keep in shape. As a result, while working as a sociologist, he spent a lot of spare time at Stagg Field helping younger runners. When the job of track coach at the U. of C. opened up in the late 1940s, Ted took it. He would have a major influence on the development of track and field in the United States, because he opened the university's facilities to out-of-college athletes, founding the University of Chicago Track Club (UCTC). Although Ted died in 1985, that club remains active today.

Ted's training system was one step up in sophistication from those of my coaches at Carleton. He employed more speedwork and prescribed somewhat more miles, although not that many more miles; otherwise I would have been unable to handle the load. Mark that as one more secret to improving as a masters runner. At least when you are preparing for a particular event, whether track meet or road race, you need to gradually increase the degree and difficulty of your training over a period of weeks and months and sometimes even years. (A key word in that sentence is "gradually.") One year out of college, I probably doubled my mileage from 15 miles a week to near 30 miles a week. Most of those miles were run at a faster pace. Fortunately, Ted's workouts were only one notch up in difficulty from those of my Carleton coaches. If the jump had been much higher, I might have been unable to make it.

These extra miles were run most frequently with Lawton Lamb Jr., who was working as a printing salesman for his father, Lawton Lamb Sr. Lawton

> You need to gradually increase the degree and difficulty of your training over a period of weeks and months and sometimes even years.

usually trained in faded green clothes. His wife had thrown a green sweat suit into the wash with most of his other clothes, and the color had in-

> Although I did not yet realize it, I was being pulled up to the next level of competition.

fected everything he owned. Particularly on days when Lawton had speedwork scheduled, I would wait for him to show up at Stagg Field after work. By that time, it would be dark and cold, particularly toward the end of the cross-country season before we moved inside to the relative comfort of the indoor track.

Ted moved a ticket booth from the Stagg era onto the infield grass to protect him from the cold. Lawton and I would run quarter-mile repeats, as many as a dozen, walking or jogging between each fast 440. Because this was cross-country season, we would run on the grass inside the track's concrete curb. Ted would time each lap, using a flashlight so he could read the numbers. His disembodied voice would echo from the ticket booth: "Sixty-five, sixty-six, sixty-. . . ." Enough light spilled into the stadium from surrounding streetlights so Lawton and I could almost see where we were stepping. Somehow we never tripped or injured ourselves. Perhaps the soft grass surface protected us, although we would wear a rut inside the track by the end of fall.

Those were magical moments for me: training with green-clad Lawton Lamb and others at the University of Chicago. Although I did not yet realize it, I was being pulled up to the next level of competition. At the end of the school year, I traveled to St. Louis to run the 10,000 meters at the National AAU Championships, finishing fifth. The following fall, the UCTC competed in the National AAU Cross-Country Championships in Philadelphia. In addition to Walt Deike, Lawton Lamb, Jim Flynn, and I, we had on our team Phil Coleman, who would make the Olympic team in the 3000-meter steeplechase in 1956 and 1960. I placed 11th, third on the team behind Phil and Walt. The UCTC team finished second to the much-favored New York Athletic Club with its collection of Olympians, including Olympic gold medalist Horace Ashenfelter and an athlete

IMPROVING YOUR TRAINING

When I moved from Carleton to the University of Chicago, I made a major jump in ability, partly because I found faster training companions, but also because I followed a somewhat more sophisticated training program. If you want to improve as a masters runner, you need to improve your training.

Coach Ted Haydon, like many coaches from that era, was a disciple of Billy Hayes, whose teams at Indiana University had won a series of cross-country titles in the 1930s and 1940s, featuring runners like Don Lash and Fred Wilt. Coach Hayes balanced overdistance with underdistance, sprinkling speedwork into the mixture.

Distance runners coached by Ted Haydon usually had a main event (such as the mile), but trained for and raced 1 week at that distance, then shifted week-to-week to distances above (2 miles) and below (880). Thus, in a 5-week period, your training focus would be: (1) mile, (2) 880, (3) mile, (4) 2-mile, (5) mile. This prevented boredom caused by running the same workouts and races week after week. I used a similar approach while coaching high-school runners in the early 1990s, and it certainly would work for masters runners, too. In workouts featuring fast repeats, Ted had runners walk until rested. As they improved in conditioning, they would cut

who later would coach me, Fred Wilt. We missed beating the NYAC by only three points. My accomplishments in those two meets would be an important factor in my next step up as a runner.

SPEEDWORK SPELLS SUCCESS

Our semivictorious team returned to Chicago by train, and I reported for 2 years' duty with the U.S. Army. The Korean War had ended, but men still were subject to the draft. The Army sent me in November to Camp Chaffee, Arkansas, for basic training. In May, having done next to no running for the previous 5 months, I climbed aboard a troop ship bound for Europe. I was assigned to an ordnance battalion and later a tank company in Kitzingen, Germany, and even-the rest time, either by walking less or jogging between repeats. Here's how the schedule looked for a miler on Ted's team.

Monday—Overdistance: 1½ miles, or 50 percent more than your race distance. Done flat-out: 90 percent of maximum

Tuesday—Speedwork: 4 to 6 × 440. Faster than race pace

Wednesday—2 or 3 × 880 at race pace

Thursday—Speedwork: 6 to 8 × 220

Friday—Rest or easy jogging: to get ready for Saturday's race

Saturday—Competition: Race 1 mile

Sunday—Rest: to recover from Saturday's race

Because we warmed up with a mile or two and some quick sprints before the core workout and cooled down with another mile, I was covering more distance than I had at Carleton—though not as much as I would in another year or two. I also was doing more speedwork. Yes, you do need to increase quantity and quality of your training if you want to improve as a masters runner. But any steps you take should be simple and well-considered.

tually transferred to Seventh Army Headquarters near Stuttgart. My next step up in ability and knowledge would be managed by an athlete I had run against in college: Frank McBride.

After graduation from South Dakota State, Frank entered the Army as an ROTC (Reserve Officers Training Corps) officer. The Army shipped Lieutenant McBride to West Berlin to serve as a track coach. Competition in the Army began at the company level. If you ran well, you moved up to a battalion, then a division team. This allowed you to go on TDY (temporary duty) and avoid the tedious chores of regular Army life. Because of my successes in national competition (track and cross-country) just before entering the Army, I eventually qualified for time off-duty, several hours at the end of each day, to train for the Olympics. Frank and I renewed our friendship when the First

Division team for which I had qualified traveled to Berlin to compete against a team he coached. Coincidentally, one of my teammates was Palmer "Pete" Retzlaff, a former teammate of Frank's at South Dakota State, later a tight end and general manager of the Philadelphia Eagles.

That summer, I competed in Athens, Greece, at the CISM (*Conseil International du Sport Militaire*) Championships. Frank McBride served as head coach. I placed second in the 3000-meter steeplechase in 1955 and third the following year in Berlin. Discharged from the service, Frank remained in Europe as a Department of the Army civilian sports consultant, transferred to Stuttgart where I was then stationed. Also stationed in Stuttgart during the winter of 1955–56 was Dean Thackwray, a New Englander who became my regular training partner. Almost weekly Dean and I ran at the VfB Stuttgart sports club's track with Stefan Lupfert, the German indoor 3000-meter champion. Again, I had the opportunity to train with athletes who could push me in practice. Dean returned to the United States in April to run the Boston Marathon, eventually qualifying for the U.S. team that competed in the 1956 Olympic Games in Melbourne, Australia.

I have vivid memories from the previous summer of 1955, attending a track meet in Fürth, a suburb of Nürnberg, where I was training with the Army team. Several of my teammates had been invited to run in the meet, but I was not yet up to that level. Running the 5000 meters that evening was Emil Zatopek of Czechoslovakia, arguably the greatest distance runner of the 20th century. Paavo Nurmi, Lasse Viren, and Haile Gebrselassie all have their supporters, but it is hard to argue with Zatopek's accomplishments. At the 1952 Olympic Games, he won gold medals in the 5000 meters, 10,000 meters, and marathon. Between 1948 and 1954, he won 38 consecutive 10,000-meter races. During his career, Zatopek set 18 world records.

I crowded close to the railing to get the best possible view of the Czech star, whose main rival that evening was Hans Laufer of Germany (himself good enough to place fourth in the Olympic 3000-meter steeplechase a year later). Zatopek was famous for his ungainly style, his arms thrashing wildly, his face contorted in agony. Yet beneath the waist, he was all business, his legs propelling him swiftly around the track.

Leaning over the railing, I wondered what it would take to be able to race the great Zatopek. Even to be lapped by him would be an honor. But my best times during the summer of 1955 were 15:40 for the 5000 meters, 9:03 for the 3000 meters. With times that slow, I could never hope to be more than a spectator to greatness.

One year later, it was I in that same track meet racing Laufer. Zatopek did not reappear, and I got beat by Laufer, but I had moved from spectator to competitor. My times that summer of 1956 dropped to 14:43.6 in the 5000, 8:33.8 in the 3000.

What was the difference? Interval training.

Long runs in the *Schwarzwald* (or Black Forest) with Dean Thackwray and workouts on the track with Stefan Lupfert certainly contributed to my next step up in ability, but I also learned from Frank McBride, who studied the interval training methods of the German coach Waldemar Gerschler. Gerschler's prize runner had been Rudolf Harbig, who set a world 800 record of 1:46.6 in 1939, finally broken by Roger Moens (1:45.7) in 1955. (Harbig was killed serving in the German Army during World War II.)

Few coaches back home had yet discovered Gerschler, whose unique version of speedwork featured fast repeats of various distances from 200 to 1000 meters with short intervals between where the athlete jogged at a semifast pace that maintained his heart rate at a high level until starting the next fast repeat. The fast repeats typically were slower than those I had done with Lawton Lamb, but the intervals between were done more quickly at a fast jogging pace, typically 8:00 per mile.

After a winter of hard training, I reported in the spring with approximately 80 other Army runners identified as having Olympic potential to a training camp in Nürnberg. One distance runner on our squad was Gar Williams, who a decade later would win a National AAU Marathon Championship. Other teammates included Ira Murchison, a gold medalist on the 4 × 100 relay team at the 1956 Olympics, and Dickie Howard, bronze medalist in the 400-meter hurdles at the 1960 Olympics. We were a fairly talented bunch, plus we had a good coach in Frank McBride.

We trained on several tracks in a sports complex near the square where Hitler had harangued the Nazi Party Congress in 1934, an

---

THE GERMAN METHOD

During the winter of 1955–56, Dean Thackwray and I trained as often as possible on the track of the VfB Stuttgart sports club with that club's distance runners, the fastest being Stefan Lupfert, the German indoor 3000-meter champion. I still possess a chart of my workouts from that period. A typical workout was on March 10, 1956: 3 miles warmup; 10 × 400 in 73.5; 1 mile cooldown.

That doesn't sound that difficult for a runner of Lupfert's ability, or even for Dean and me at that point. (I probably ran 400 repeats 5 or 10 seconds faster at Carleton and the University of Chicago.) The difference—and the secret of the German method—was the interval between each fast repetition. This was the training approach of Waldemar Gerschler: Closely control the interval so that the runner's heart rate remained high between each fast repetition. We "jogged" the 400 interval between in just under 2 minutes, allowing some recovery, but not too much rest. We probably ran a 10 × 400 workout with 400 between (20 laps, 5 miles total) in less than half an hour.

Later, after I returned to Chicago, some of my training partners would complain that we were running too slow—until they got to about the sixth or seventh repetition. If they had mistakenly sprinted ahead of me during the early repeats, they often would fail to finish the workout. As described in my book *Run Fast*, Gerschler's interval training included five variables.

1. **Distance.** How far you run each repetition

2. **Interval.** How long you rest during each interval

3. **Repetitions.** How many times you run the distance

4. **Pace.** How fast you run during the distance

5. **Rest.** What you do during the interval

event immortalized in *Triumph of the Will* by filmmaker Leni Riefenstahl. (Riefenstahl, who died recently at the age of 101, also directed *Olympia,* the documentary of the 1936 Olympic Games in Berlin.) We drove through that square every day, barely mindful of

---

Many runners—and even some book authors—mistakenly talk about running fast "intervals," when they really mean fast "repetitions." The "interval" is what goes on between the fast runs, and Gerschler wanted this element tightly controlled. An interval could be 100, 200, 300 meters, or more. It could involve walking or jogging. Some coaches and runners even use heart monitors to dictate when to start running fast again. The important point is that you know precisely your training plan for the workout before you execute it. Ah, yes: so very German! Here are some variations from my training log from that period during the spring of 1956 when I was training in Nürnberg under Frank McBride getting ready for the Olympic trials.

50 × 100, 100 between

30 × 200, 200 between

17 × 400, 400 between

5 × (400, 300, 200, 100), 200 between

10 × (500, 100), 300 and 100 between

8 × (600, 200), 200 between

Many of the workouts, which seem strange even to me today, were done mainly for variety, since I was doing speedwork every day. It kept me from getting bored by not repeating the same workout. To explain, the "10 × (500, 100), 300 and 100 between" workout could better be described as: 500 fast, 300 rest, 100 fast, 100 rest—then repeat everything 10 times.

The German method worked, allowing me to chop a full minute off my 5000 time in the space of a year. But it also can lead to overtraining, particularly if you do speedwork day after day. Later in my career, when I tried to use interval training for the marathon, I learned that modifications were necessary.

its historical significance. I was focused on applying the new interval training methods of Gerschler. I ran interval workouts on the track nearly every day. One day I ran 200s, another day 400s; sometimes I mixed distances, alternating between 600s and 200s, 200 jogs between. I combined interval workouts with long runs, training twice daily, running 60 to 70 miles a week. I also ran hurdles, since my main event was the steeplechase. The combination of distance and speed allowed me to chop a full minute off my best time for 5000 meters in 1 year. My times at other distances improved similarly and significantly.

At no other period in my running career did I achieve such a level of improvement, and it was all due to interval training—or so I thought.

Fast training, thus, is the third secret for success as a masters runner. And it could be the most important secret. Long-distance running at relatively slow paces can only carry you so far. If you want to improve, you need to add speedwork. Interestingly, 71 percent of the approximately 500 masters runners who responded to my online questionnaire do just that.

Alas, Frank McBride and I learned another lesson, although it would be several more years before either of us fully understood it. Too much speedwork can result in overtraining and reduced success. At the beginning of my training program, when I was still running with Dean Thackwray and Stefan Lupfert, I began with a workout of 10 × 400 meters in 70 seconds, jogging 400 in 2 minutes for the interval between. Each week, I would add one more quarter and drop the average time by 1 second. I continued this seemingly logical progression when I moved from Stuttgart to Nürnberg. My top workout before the Army team departed for California and the Olympic trials was 17 × 400, averaging 62.8. The following week, I ran a 10,000 in a trial to select the 22 runners making the team to California and cranked out 75-second laps almost without effort, setting a personal record of 31:06.5. The time seems ordinary to me now, but this was during an era of cinder rather than all-weather tracks, when many of us were still figuring out how to train. It was the second fastest time by an American that Olympic year.

Unfortunately, I never did make that Olympic team. I had been burning the candle at both ends. I learned that you can progress an interval workout by doing more repeats each week, or running those repeats faster. But you cannot do both!

Focused on a false goal of running 20 × 400 meters in 60 seconds, I had overlooked the fact that my real goal should have been to succeed at the Olympic trials. I had been blindsided by my ambition and unwillingness to modify a training schedule that was just too tough. Thus, the fourth secret of success as a masters runner: Pick your goals carefully, but don't pick overly ambitious goals. If you begin to struggle following a preconceived training schedule, modify it.

After arriving in California, I tried to resume training at the same level. I crashed badly after attempting an 18 × 400 workout in California, failing to allow for my fatigue from having flown halfway around the world. (This was before the jet era.) My workouts suffered. My performances sagged. I came down with some breathing problems that never did get properly diagnosed. I was badly overtrained. In the Olympic trials for 10,000 meters in Bakersfield, I ran even with Max Truex for 4 miles, then faded, finishing in the top 10, but with a time too embarrassing to report. I returned to Europe and after a brief period of rest recovered and set personal records in the steeplechase and 5000 racing in Finland, but I missed the message that interval training was no cure-all, that intensive doses of speedwork could do you as much harm as good. McBride and Gerschler had allowed me to move to the next level, but that level was not high enough to fulfill my ambitions. I spent the next 4 years hoping that more miles combined with daily doses of speedwork was the secret of success. It was not. I was worshipping the wrong god. Only when I modified my training, retaining some speedwork, but blending it with steady distance running, was I able to progress once again.

BLENDING SPEED AND DISTANCE

That progress came under the direction of Fred Wilt, a 1948 and 1952 Olympian who had competed for Indiana University and later the New York Athletic Club while working as an FBI agent. Toward the end of the 1950s, the FBI assigned Fred to an office in Lafayette, Indiana. (After leaving the Bureau, Fred would become women's coach at Purdue University.) Fred continued to train into his forties and fifties, but no longer raced competitively. Like Ted Haydon, he also played around with the hammer and became as knowledgeable about field events as distance events. In his spare time, he coached a few top athletes, including Ollan Cassell, a member of the 4 × 400 relay team that won the gold medal at the 1964 Olympic Games and later executive director of the U.S. Track and Field Federation.

Fred also coached Buddy Edelen, who was living and working in England. Buddy set a world marathon record of 2:14:28 in 1963, so I was very much the lesser of the two distance runners Fred coached by mail. Buddy and I each filled out diary sheets of our daily workouts, mailing them to Fred at the end of the week. Fred would critique our training, underlining our comments, adding his own in red pen, and mail the sheets right back.

Fred taught me how to blend speedwork with long runs, balancing the two ingredients that can assure success whether you are an open or masters runner. But I probably learned as much from him about managing time and fitting training into a busy lifestyle. Fred and his wife, Ellie, had three girls, who absorbed a lot of love and affection. Plus he was working a full-time job with the FBI and did not have the luxury of devoting 2 or 3 hours to his running daily. He found ways to train efficiently instead.

One workout I saw him do on several occasions was to go to the high-school track near his Lafayette home, run eight laps (or 2 miles), then head home. The first four laps he did at a jog: his warmup. Then without stopping, Fred would run a fast 200, jog 200, then repeat that three more times. In other words: 4 × 200. His cooldown was the final jogging 200 after the last fast repeat. Very quick. Very efficient. Given Fred's ability, he could do that 2-mile workout in 15 minutes and be home for dinner with Ellie and the girls. I still use a variation of this workout on occasions when I am pressed for time.

Consider this as the fifth secret for success as a masters runner:

Manage your time properly. Most important, don't waste time. Runners who have jobs, families, and other commitments can't spend their day focused entirely on their training as do professional runners.

Nevertheless, efficiency has its limits. You can't challenge for victory in the Boston Marathon with 15-minute workouts. Even more than making the Olympic team in 1964, winning Boston became my goal, my obsession. Fred determined the direction of my training, specifically the pattern of blending speed and distance that I still use today in directing runners of all ages and abilities who want to compete in 26-mile 385-yard races.

The key Wilt distance workouts were on Sundays and Wednesdays. At peak training, I ran 20 to 23 miles each Sunday. Each Wednesday, I ran 13 to 16 miles, approximately two-thirds of the longer distance. If you check my marathon training programs online or in my book, *Marathon: The Ultimate Training Guide,* you will recognize the pattern of a long run on the weekend and what I describe as a "sorta-long" run in the middle of the week.

On several other days of the week, I ran speedwork. Fred liked 400-meter repeats, classic interval training à la Gerschler—but not every day of the week. He also recommended 100-meter sprints, feeling that marathon runners needed to have the ability to run fast as well as run long. I ran twice daily, my second workout usually being an easy run of 4 to 8 miles. "Easy" for me back then was a 6:00- to 7:00-mile pace. At peak I covered more than 100 miles a week.

That training allowed me to finish fifth (first American) at Boston in 1964. I ran my fastest road race between 1963 and 1965 with Fred's assistance, but by then I was in my mid-thirties with a realization that the next generation of runners was younger and faster and capable of times better than even Buddy Edelen. The American distance running scene was still a half-generation away with Frank Shorter, Bill Rodgers, Alberto Salazar, and Joan Benoit, but in 1965, I stopped mailing diary sheets to Fred. With no more Olympic goals, I

> Even more than making the Olympic team, winning Boston became my goal, my obsession.

ACHIEVING PEAK PERFORMANCE

My greatest success as an elite runner came under the direction of Fred Wilt, who coached me by mail between 1963 and 1965. Fred blended high mileage and quick speedwork with easy recovery days—although as you will see by examining the schedule that follows, "easy" back then meant a run of a dozen miles at a comfortable pace in the afternoon after 6 miles in the morning!

Perhaps Fred's greatest contribution, however, was providing me with a direction, peace of mind, and the knowledge that I was training at an appropriate level to achieve my goals. By then, I already knew what worked for me, but Fred reinforced what I knew, providing positive feedback. If I needed a push, he gave it. If I needed to be reined back, he pulled back. Fred was providing Buddy Edelen with similar input at the same time, one reason for Buddy's success in running a world-record marathon in 1963. Just as an attorney who represents himself in court is said to have a fool for a client, runners who coach themselves also can come up short. It helps to have a coach.

During this period, I traveled frequently on assignment for magazines as diverse as *Good Housekeeping* and *Sports Illustrated,* so my workouts usually varied from week to week. Following is a somewhat typical 8 days from March 1964.

Sunday—Long run: 20 miles in just over 2 hours (a 6:00-mile pace)

cut my training in half, though I still continued to run for enjoyment. I did not realize that in a half-dozen years and at the age of 40, I would be motivated to reevaluate my running goals and resume the tough training necessary for success as a masters runner.

A CHALLENGING GOAL

At the start of 1972, having turned 40 the previous summer, I set as my goal not any masters competition, not even the trip to Europe David Pain was planning for later that year, but rather qualifying for

Monday—Easy day: 6 miles in morning; 12 in afternoon

Tuesday—Speedwork: 6 miles in morning; 27 × 440 in evening (75 seconds per 440, 30-second jog between)

Wednesday—Sorta-long run: 10 easy miles in morning; 15 miles in afternoon in 1:40:00 (a 6:45 pace)

Thursday—Speedwork: 11 easy miles in morning; 110s and 220s in afternoon at race pace, walking or jogging between (almost a fartlek workout on track)

Friday—Recovery: 6 easy miles in morning

Saturday—Recovery: 6 easy miles in morning

Sunday—Race: 1st in Windy City Marathon: 2:35:04

Given the fact that I usually prescribe a 3-week taper, most runners today would consider it strange that I would run 110 miles the week before a race. Actually, I considered Windy City more a controlled time trial than serious competition. I cruised most of the race well behind the leaders and only moved in front with 3 miles to go. One month later at Boston, I ran a personal record of 2:21:55, a pace 30 seconds faster per mile.

Few runners could survive this level of training—and I didn't always survive—but the blend of distance, speed, and recovery still can work for runners trying to achieve peak performance, regardless of their age.

the Olympic trials in the marathon. Prior to 1972, anyone could compete in the marathon trials, which for many years had been the exclusive property of Boston and Yonkers. For most of the century, there existed only a handful of marathons in the United States, and those two were the most prestigious. But during the 1960s, road running, once almost exclusively a New England sport, began to spread westward into the rest of the United States. One of the two marathon trials in 1964 was in Culver City, California. In 1968, a single trial was held at high altitude in Alamosa, Colorado, because the Olympic Games were in Mexico City at a similar altitude. For the 1972 trials, the AAU long-distance running committee chose Eugene, Oregon, and for the first time set a qualifying standard for entry.

> Instead of training being a means to an end, it often becomes the end itself.

To enter the trials, men needed to have run a 2:30 marathon the previous year. (There were no Olympic trials in the marathon for women, because the women's marathon did not get added to the Olympic schedule until 1984.)

That time of 2:30 seemed well within my grasp, but I knew I would have to train hard to achieve it. I had no desire to mimic the twice-a-day and 100-miles-a-week routine that had brought me success under Fred Wilt. By then I was a masters runner and had explored nearly every training option imaginable. Instead of training being a means to an end, it often became the end itself. The goal of achieving a fast time offered an excuse to train hard and fast, and that sounded like fun.

I decided to train for the marathon by doing something different. That becomes the sixth secret if you want to achieve success as a masters runner: Change your training habits. If your previous focus has been on long runs and marathon competition, shift to 5-K and 10-K races. Cut back on your total miles, but increase the pace of your workouts. If you want to shift upward in distance, then cut back on speedwork and start doing longer workouts at a slower pace. And between running long and running fast, you need a third period where you do very little running to both recover from injuries and the malaise that comes when you run the same workouts year after year after year. Separating your training into periods of speed, distance, and recovery is what today's coaches refer to as periodization.

Fortunately, I had just come through a long period—6 years, in fact—when I had not taken my training too seriously. Even my first masters race at the 1971 National AAU Championships in San Diego had been run with minimal training. But by the following year, my motivation was high for a return to glory. That is the seventh secret for success as a masters runner: Keep running, but don't be afraid to take time off from competition. A good time to do this is the last year or two before you move up to a new age group.

In 1964, Rose and I had moved our family to Michigan City, Indiana, a small town of about 35,000 inhabitants 55 miles around the bottom of Lake Michigan from Chicago. We chose the Michigan City area partly because it was a small town. This was the 1960s, and while Michigan City had most of the same urban problems as Chicago, being smaller, its problems somehow seemed more manageable. Admittedly, the main reason for our move was real estate: location, location, location. In Long Beach, a lakefront suburb of Michigan City, we could afford a house overlooking the lake that would have been prohibitively expensive anywhere in the city of Chicago or its suburbs. In Chicago, I spent too much time training on tracks or pavement. Long Beach offered numerous low-traffic roads and trails through the woods. I had chosen as my place of residence a long-distance runner's paradise, and I still live there today.

Our home on Lake Shore Drive was little more than a mile from the Michigan state line, about 6 minutes of running for me back then. Seven miles northeast along the lakefront was New Buffalo, Michigan, now a magnet for Chicagoans with second homes, then a sleepy village that nobody had heard of. Between Long Beach and New Buffalo were a string of lakefront communities: Shoreland Hills, Duneland Beach, Michiana, Michiana Shores, and Grand Beach. A corridor about a half-mile wide between the lake and US-12 became the focus of my training runs, much of the corridor wooded with often hilly trails winding in all directions. It became the mission of training partner Steve Kearney and me to identify a course connecting Long Beach and New Buffalo stepping on as little pavement as possible.

Steve was a senior at Chesterton High School when we first met. He spent 4 years running track and cross-country at Ball State University, then returned to teach mathematics and coach track at his former high school. It took several years during that period for Steve and me to develop a course that was impossible to measure, but I judged to be about 13.5 miles based on how long it took to run it. During one of our runs, we got lost in the woods in Grand Beach and exited a trail into someone's backyard. Two angry-looking men in dark suits moved toward us. The backyard and house belonged to Chicago Mayor Richard J. Daley, father of the current mayor.

A SPECIAL TRAINING COURSE

The 13.5-mile course Steve and I finally developed began and ended with a mile plus of pavement on Lake Shore Drive, an unavoidable negative in one respect, except since I had each quarter-mile measured, it allowed me to check my pace both at the start and finish of each workout. Just past 1 mile heading north, the course turned diagonally right and crossed from Indiana into Michigan, climbing a short but steep hill. The course covered another half-mile or so of pavement along the state line before another hill, short but steep up and down. Next, the course crossed a creek and turned northward onto a horse path paralleling that creek. Except after a rain, the horse trail was soft, uneven, winding, and rolling, a nice change of surface, constant change being the most important attribute of the 13.5-mile course.

Coming off the trail, the course shifted to a gravel road (paved some years later), then onto a golf course at 3 miles, the last marker where I could catch a split to figure out approximately how fast I was running. After several minutes of smooth fairway running, the course moved onto trails that bordered a marsh. Sometimes they were muddy, sometimes firm. Then back into the woods, up a sandy hill where I once nearly stepped on a rattlesnake. (I swear I changed stride midair and floated over his coiled body.) Then a roller-coaster ride featuring direction and elevation changes before the course dropped down to the beach, which could be fast or slow depending on recent wave action.

Within a mile, the course reached the edge of New Buffalo, moving up a sandy hill to loop through a subdivision, then back into the woods before bursting out to US-12 heading back south next to the (now Amtrak) railroad tracks. Rocks from the roadbed often made the trail beside the tracks tricky to run, so I usually moved to the shoulder of the road. But quickly I was back on a smoother,

wooded trail that con-
nected soon with the path
beside the marsh I had
left 2 or 3 miles earlier.

> Keep running, but don't be afraid to take time off from competition.

I didn't know exactly
how far I had run at this point and didn't care. Returning across the
golf course, I reached 3-miles-to-go where I could monitor my pace
again. During the spring of 1972, I usually ran this course very fast,
probably near 90 percent of maximum, almost full effort. I ran the
course every third or fourth day. Over a period of weeks, I tried to
do each 13.5-miler somewhat faster than the one before, finally
peaking with a time under 1:15:00, a pace fast enough to win most
area races near that distance, even against open competition.

The eighth secret of success for masters runners is to find trails
like mine for your hardest workouts. Choose bouncy surfaces like
that of a golf course to protect against injury, but don't totally
abandon pavement. Vary your surfaces. Vary your paces. And when-
ever possible, pick locales pleasing to the eye.

After running as fast as I conceived possible on my 13.5-mile
course, I added 4 more miles at the start of the run, crossing a different golf course and around a lake on a trail that at one point sent
me crashing through bramble bushes that ripped my legs, speckling
them with blood. My new course was close to 17 miles, which
meant I could slow somewhat and not compare times with previous
13.5-milers. And after I maxed out on that course, I added 3 more
miles in the town of New Buffalo, reaching 20 miles. Or pretty close
to it. I was only able to complete two 20-milers in June before my
planned marathon.

I chose The Longest Day Marathon in Brookings, South Dakota.
The race got its name because it was held on or near June 21, the
longest day of the year. Some years later, the race directors sought
cooler weather and moved their marathon to earlier in the spring, yet
retained the name "Longest Day" for reasons I still don't understand.
I chose the race partly because of its flat course, but more because
our two sons, Kevin and David, were going on a Boy Scout trip to
South Dakota. I've always tried to blend my running with a family

life. But the late-spring marathon also gave me more time to get in shape to achieve my goal: qualify for the Olympic marathon trials. The trials actually were only a few weeks after my race, but I was less interested in running them than in qualifying for them.

One flaw in my plan was that I hadn't anticipated the weather I would encounter in Brookings. The temperature at the start was 62

PLUNGING THROUGH THE WOODS

Most effective training programs provide some form of progression. You run progressively more miles in individual workouts and in training weeks. This is the approach I take in coaching first-time marathoners, increasing the weekend long runs from 6 to 20 miles, the weekly mileage from 15 to 40. More experienced runners often train by keeping their mileage constant, or even decreasing it, but running at a faster pace.

Doing both—progressing with speed and distance—can be tricky and lead to injury or overtraining, but I succeeded with this approach during the spring of 1972 as I prepared for the Longest Day Marathon.

I did my hardest training on a 13.5-mile course between Long Beach, Indiana and New Buffalo, Michigan. I ran this course every second or third day, faster each time. My goal was to run 1:15, about a 5:45 pace. In the space of a month, I ran the course 10 times before achieving the goal. Then I lengthened the course to 17 miles, slowed my pace somewhat, and set a new goal at 1:42, about a 6:00 pace. I ran that course six times in the next 3 weeks. That goal achieved, I upped the distance to 20 miles with a goal of 2 hours, also a 6:00 pace. Here is the progression.

April 14: 13.5 miles, untimed

April 18: 13.5 miles, 1:35

April 20: 13.5 miles, 1:28

April 24: 13.5 miles, 1:40 (stiff afterward)

May 1: 13.5 miles, 1:24:15

May 3: 13.5 miles, 1:20:40

with humidity at 78 percent, but more a problem were winds gusting between 15 and 25 miles per hour. The flat plain provided no windbreaks. The course was a square with a tail: four 6-mile straightaways, then runners headed toward an athletic field to run the last half-mile on a track.

The ninth secret of masters running success is to have flexible

---

May 5: 13.5 miles, 1:18:50

May 10: 13.5 miles, 1:17:28

May 12: 13.5 miles, 1:17:00

May 16: 13.5 miles, 1:14:52

May 19: 17 miles, 2:00:30

May 23: 13.5 miles, 1:49:00 (easy)

May 26: 17 miles, 1:58:10

May 30: 17 miles, 1:50:00

June 1: 17 miles, 1:58:15 (fatigued)

June 4: 17 miles, 1:47:38

June 6: 17 miles, 1:40:50

June 8: 20 miles, 2:44:30

June 10: 20 miles, 2:19:05

June 18: Longest Day Marathon; 1st, 2:37:24

Does this behavior now seem obsessive? Yes, but it achieved results. Because of an injury I suffered when thrown from a horse, I never did run my 20-mile course faster than 2 hours, but I met almost all my competitive goals that summer, the climax coming during David Pain's European tour for masters. That I was able to train at such intensity may partially have been because I trained on forgiving surfaces. Plunging through the woods can often be a very intelligent means to train. Also, it's a lot more fun.

goals. Take each race for what it gives you. Don't let the weather defeat you, even if it means you may run slower than ex-

> Sometimes we need to fail before being allowed to succeed.

pected. Define your own degree of victory.

My main rival was a runner who boasted a marathon best of 2:26; he moved quickly into the lead along the first straightaway with the wind beating us from over our left shoulders. Wise about marathon strategy, I ran conservatively, trying to stay near the 5:45-mile pace that would allow me to achieve my 2:30 goal. Reaching a crossroad at about 6 miles, we turned left into the wind. I held pace and soon passed my rival, who was struggling because of the weather.

Near 12 miles, the course turned left again, providing relief. The wind, now blowing off my right shoulder, seemed manageable. I held pace through 18 miles and turned left again onto a final 6-mile straightaway where I would have the wind at my back. I figured I could fly and beat my goal time with minutes to spare.

Alas, I had not counted on the rising heat and a sun beating relentlessly on my head. By now, the temperature probably was in the 70s. I still held pace, but I could feel my body temperature rising. With the wind at my back, I now felt no cooling effect from it. I knew I needed a time cushion for when I turned upwind again in the 25th mile, but I could not get it. Despite reaching 24 miles on pace, I was toast. My goal was unattainable. Nobody was in sight behind, reducing my motivation to push hard. (The second place runner finished more than 7 minutes back.) Incredibly, it took me 4:40 to run the last half-mile on the track. Half-mile, not mile! My winning time was 2:37:24. My time established a course record. I won the race overall, but my time also was a masters record that went unbroken until 1999 by Steve Wilson. He also won the 2004 race in 2:32.37.

EASY RIDER

I failed to achieve an Olympic trials qualifying time, but I consider Longest Day, given the conditions, one of my best marathons.

It certainly proved the soundness of the admittedly bizarre training program that led to that race: the progressive series of longer and faster runs that peaked at 20 miles. All my training programs today in books and on the Internet for novice, intermediate, and advanced runners feature a steady progression in long-run distance. But the more important message for masters runners is that once you understand the principles of training, you can design your own schedules to suit your specific needs and interests. Certainly, the scenic beauty of my courses made running hard on them more tolerable.

Immediately after the race with my two sons in tow, we joined their Boy Scout troop. The troop planned to spend a week camping and horseback riding in the wilderness. I never had been on a horse before, nor did I realize that the horse assigned to me was flighty. The cowboy in charge offered no instruction, figuring we were all seasoned riders. I mounted the horse, and it immediately bucked me off.

I landed uninjured and immediately remounted the horse, since that's what you're supposed to do when thrown, plus I wanted to regain as much of my dignity as possible. The horse took off at a flat-out sprint that ended in 200 meters when he flipped me again. This time I did not get up so quickly. I lay on the ground dazed, other fathers and scouts and my two worried sons hovering over me. I could not breathe. I could not move. This was before Christopher Reeve's horseback injury that left him paralyzed for life, but for a moment, I wondered if I would run another marathon again, much less win one. I soon regained my composure and was helped off the ground and taken to a hospital. Complicating my problem was the fact that I had just run a marathon, meaning every muscle in my body should have been sore even without falling off a horse.

As I lay in the hospital bed, a nurse approached carrying a clipboard. She wanted to know my name, my address, my occupation. I told her, "writer."

I watched the nurse as she wrote the information on her clipboard. She spelled it: r-i-d-e-r. The nurse apparently thought I was in town with some rodeo.

Within a day I was out of the hospital and back with the Boy

Scouts, although I never again attempted to mount a horse. It was several weeks after our return home before I could resume running—and at a much slower pace than my flat-out distance workouts of the spring.

Then something happened that provides the tenth and final secret of success for masters runners. Toward the end of August, I climbed on a plane bound for Europe to participate in David Pain's 1972 masters tour. Because of the enforced rest, I was seriously undertrained and nervous about how I would fare against some of the world's best masters. Within 4 days, I ran three of the best races of my life in the 3000-meter steeplechase, 5000, and 10,000, times almost as fast as when I was a younger runner.

It was the combination of extremely hard training followed by an appropriate amount of rest that brought me to the height of my glory. Rest, as long as you know when to rest, can be the most important ingredient of any training program. Sometimes you get lucky and get bucked off a horse before you train too hard.

Over the next several years, armed with my newfound knowledge, I ran some of the best races of my life, climaxed by winning the 3000-meter steeplechase at the World Masters Championships in Toronto at age 44. My time was only 5 seconds slower than my personal record from 2 decades before. If only I had known in my twenties what I knew in my forties, I might have turned most of my failures into successes. But events often work out for the best. Sometimes we need to fail before being allowed to succeed. Having failed while knowing I could do better was part of the motivation that allowed me to excel as a masters runner.

SECRETS OF MASTERS SUCCESS

Here are the secrets that took me decades to learn. They can make you a better masters runner in a much shorter period of time.

1. **Be consistent.** You need to train year-round. Masters runners particularly don't need to train every day, since occasional and well-planned rest days can contribute to fitness, but you

need to train most days. Vitally important: You need to avoid long periods when you fail to run.

2. **Find good training partners.** It doesn't matter whether they are younger or older than you, somewhat slower or somewhat faster, or which sex. You can push yourself harder in workouts running with someone near your equal in ability.

3. **Run fast.** Include speedwork in your mix of training. Long-distance running at relatively slow paces can only carry you so far. If you want to improve, you need to also run fast.

4. **Pick achievable goals.** Focusing on too lofty a goal can get you in trouble. If you begin to struggle following a preconceived training schedule designed by yourself or your coach, modify it.

5. **Manage your time efficiently.** Most important, don't waste time. Runners who have jobs, families, and other commitments can't spend their day obsessed with their training. In other words, get a real life.

6. **Change your training habits.** Do something different. If your past focus has been distance, shift to speedwork. If a speed freak, try more long runs. And don't overlook periods when you cut your training back to near zero to relax and recover.

7. **Take breaks.** Never stop running completely, but you don't need to compete continuously. Quit racing for a while. A good time to take a break from competition is the last year or two before you move up to a new age group.

8. **Choose different surfaces.** Trails through the woods are best for your hardest workouts. Run different paces. Run up hills and down. Mostly, find areas that are scenic and where even the toughest training can be a joy.

9. **Have flexible goals.** You can't change the weather and often can't even predict it. The course may be tougher than

expected. Faster runners may or may not appear to make victory easy or unattainable. As long as you know you're a champion, don't worry what the rest of the world thinks.

10. **Don't overlook rest.** Too much or too hard training can be as bad for you as too little. Tapering works in the marathon, and it works in other races, too. Never overtrain, because undertraining will take you farther for years and years of masters running.

6 CHALLENGE

Plan Properly, Train Correctly, and Sometimes You Get It Perfectly Right

Flying home from the World Masters Championships in Hanover, Germany, in August 1979, I began to plan my campaign. The next championships would be in Christchurch, New Zealand, in January 1981, less than 18 months away. Because the masters meet was being held in the Southern Hemisphere for the first time, the dates of competition had been changed to the middle of New Zealand's summer. As a result, in Christchurch I would be 5 months short of my 50th birthday, running in the M45 age group for the third time in 5 years. Had the championships been planned for its usual time of year, I would have moved into a new age group. Presumably, I would have an easier time winning a medal in the M50 division than M45.

But that was the challenge! Who wants easy? The fact that the odds seemed stacked against me made me more determined to succeed.

My early trips to the World Masters Championships had, indeed, met with success. At the inaugural championships in Toronto in 1975, I competed in the M40 division, winning the 3000-meter steeplechase and placing third in cross-country. Two years later, I moved up an age division and won gold in the steeplechase and bronze in the marathon at the age of 46. Only in comparison with those two outings did my results in Germany seem mediocre. I placed second in both the 10,000 and steeplechase and fourth in the 5000, reasonable results for someone who at 48 was approaching the far end of his age group, but I wanted to do better than reasonable in Christchurch. And to further the challenge, I wanted to do it in the marathon, an event in which I had struggled earlier in my career.

Maybe it was a surfeit of fast-twitch muscles. I had been a miler in college, eventually getting down to 4:13.6, but it took me a while to realize that I never would see the underside of 4 minutes. I began to drift upward in distance, waiting until age 27 to run my first marathon at Boston, but my early attempts at that distance had ended in failure.

I dropped out of both the 1959 and 1960 Boston Marathons, following the strategy that had always worked well for me on the track: running with the leaders for as long as possible, then hanging on to finish. That's the strategy that earned me that personal record in the mile, but it usually doesn't work in the marathon unless you were born in Kenya's Rift Valley, and sometimes not even then. In between those two Boston failures, I had attempted the Western Hemisphere Marathon in Culver City, California. I led most of the way, got passed at 20 miles, and was sitting on the curb again 2 miles later.

When I appeared at the National AAU Marathon in Yonkers, New York, in May 1960, I was a dismal 0-3 in marathon attempts, and I came pretty close to running my record to 0-4. In its last half-dozen miles, the Yonkers course follows the Hudson River and features one hill after another, including one at 24 miles both longer and higher than Heartbreak Hill in Boston. Halfway up that hill, I was sitting on the curb again. After about 5 minutes of feeling sorry for myself, I rose and decided to hitchhike to the finish line 2 miles away. I stuck out my thumb and waited for some kind and considerate driver to offer me a ride.

And waited.

And waited.

I can't imagine that many drivers in this era cruising past a runner with a number pinned to his singlet, but this was the 60s and it was New York. Disgusted with myself and the passing drivers, I finally started running again and crossed my first marathon finish

> Even great runners sometimes make foolish mistakes.

line. Despite my pause on the curb, I still broke 3 hours, running 2:59:00.

I ran no marathons the following year, but returned to Boston in 1962 planning to run a controlled pace well back of the leaders. I cruised home in 26th, one place behind John A. Kelley, my time 2:45:21. In 1963, I followed a similar tactic and improved my place to 13th and my time to 2:36:13. That was the year that Ethiopians Abebe Bikila and Malmo Wolde led from the beginning and set course records all the way through 20 miles. Bikila had won the Olympic marathon in 1960 and would do so again in 1964. Wolde would win the Olympic title in 1968. Even great runners sometimes make foolish mistakes, and both Ethiopians struggled badly in the last half-dozen miles, Bikila fading to fifth, Wolde to 12th, one place and 1 minute ahead of me.

It was partly training, partly tactics, but by 1964 I had figured out both. At the 1964 Boston Marathon, I took 14 minutes off my previous best time, running 2:21:55, good enough for fifth overall, first American.

That was the high point of my marathon career, I thought, because there was no masters competition back in that era. At age 32 and definitely over the hill, Heartbreak as well as all others, I resigned myself to a lifetime of recreational running, even though it irritated me that only once in my marathoning career had I been able to post a time faster than 2:30. With better weather, I might have run that fast, winning the 1972 Longest Day Marathon in South Dakota, but "might have" doesn't count in sports. Most of my energy after turning 40 had been focused on shorter-distance events. For 4 years between 1973 and 1977, I didn't run a single marathon. But with the championships in Christchurch approaching, I regarded once more the race in which glory had seemed so elusive.

PLOTTING A TRAINING PROGRAM

Thanks to Fred Wilt, I knew more about training in my forties than I did in my twenties. I still ran interval workouts on the track, but integrated them with long runs, easy runs, hard medium-distance runs, and rest. Thus, while flying home from Germany with 18 months to go before Christchurch, I plotted a training program on a pad of paper. Once home, I took a large sheet of paper and drew an 18-month calendar that listed workout essentials as well as races and weekly mileage. I tacked it to the cork wall in my basement where I would see it before and after I ran. While keeping a separate diary, I also jotted notes on the calendar, most specifically mileage.

I did not want to become a mileage freak, but from my successful run at Boston 2 decades before, I knew I needed to gradually build my weekly miles to near 100. Why? Because of the advantages of what Russell H. Pate, Ph.D., director of the human performance laboratory at the University of South Carolina, describes as "cumulative caloric through-put," a term he admits he borrowed from another runner and researcher, Peter Wood, M.D.

I quoted Dr. Pate on this subject in my book *Run Fast*: "[Cumulative caloric through-put] refers to your overall caloric expenditure, your cumulative activity. You need to burn lots of calories to succeed in running, even at modest intensities." Also, by burning all those calories you get closer to your ideal running weight, which from past experience I knew for me was 138. Weigh more, and I carry too many pounds in races; weigh less, and I am more susceptible to injuries and the illnesses that come with overtraining.

During 1 month in the fall of 1979, I ran mileages of 60, 69, 61, and 71 on successive weeks. A year later, near the peak of my training, I did 100, 99, 101, and after a 66-mile week (during which I tapered for a 10-mile race), I capped off 7 days of twice-a-day training with a 111-mile week that included a fartlek workout midweek and a 20-miler on the weekend.

At the beginning of the 1980 calendar year, I wrote New Year's resolutions for various race distances between 10-K and the marathon. Utilizing some performance charts, I set my marathon goal at 2:29:10.

Among the race distance goals chosen was 1:24:59 for 25-K, a seemingly odd distance, except the Old Kent River Bank Run in Grand Rapids, Michigan, in May presented an excellent opportunity to race that distance on a fast course in predictably good weather. Despite a windy day, I beat my goal by more than a minute, clocking 1:23:52, 3 minutes faster than the American record for my age group. The time, according to one calculator, predicted a 2:27 marathon. Good news, except you still have to show up and run 26 miles that fast.

More important, I had a chance to practice my Christchurch strategy of walking through aid stations. That would allow me to drink more comfortably. On a hot day, I figured that I would gain more than I would lose by slowing to walk. And that proved true. Using my watch to judge how much those near me pulled ahead, I figured that I lost only 7 seconds each time I walked, less than a minute for the entire race. It would be impossible to determine whether this improved my final time, but I usually regained contact within a mile or two. This strategy would prove itself later at the World Masters Championships.

PUTTING IN THE MILES

Looking at my diaries for the 18-month period between Hanover and Christchurch, I maintained steady mileage. I raced more often than prudence seemingly would dictate, except I was doing little traditional speedwork on the track. Races thus became my speedwork. During the fall of 1979, I trained only once a day but kept the mileage of each workout high. Most of my workouts were on soft surfaces to soften impact and save my legs. Fortunately, I live in an area where trails through the woods are plentiful. I continued to run the 13.5-mile course from my home in Long Beach to New Buffalo, although without quite the same fanaticism as described in the previous chapter. Fartlek workouts in a nearby wooded area with looping trails provided an opportunity for speedwork. For long runs,

LEARNING TO DRINK

If there was a single tactic that allowed me to succeed in Christchurch, it was learning how to drink in a marathon. Even first-timers can now quote you chapter-and-verse on rehydration techniques, but this was 1981. David Costill had done the initial fluid replacement research for Gatorade a dozen years earlier, but not everybody had gotten the message. The Boston Athletic Association didn't add regular aid stations until 1978 and then only because Jerome Drayton, the previous year's champion, complained to the media about their lack.

If you're an elite athlete, race organizers now provide fluids in plastic bottles, easy to sip, but ordinary runners don't have that privilege. They are forced to grab cups from volunteers, thus spilling more than they drink. Gulping drinks too fast also can cause you to gag, not conducive for maintaining a steady pace. I reasoned that if I walked through each aid station, I could not only drink more fluids, but drink more comfortably.

But how much time would this cost me in the race?

I decided to experiment in a popular 25-K race in Grand Rapids, Michigan: the Old Kent River Bank Run. At each aid station, I would walk,

I ran a flat road course that was 19.5 miles long. Wiser than I was while younger, I saw no reason to find an extra half-mile to round it off at 20. Nor did I push the workout. I usually ran at a steady pace, 7:00 miles or slower.

During the fall, my best race performance was 32:16 for a 10-K in November in Dowagiac, Michigan, where I placed third overall against much younger runners. I traveled to Hawaii in December and ran 2:35:40 in the Honolulu Marathon, good considering the heat and humidity, although I faded in the closing miles and was passed by the eventual masters (M40) winner. (There was no M45 division, otherwise I would have won it.)

Winters are never easy on Midwest long-distance runners. For 3 months from December through February, cold weather and varying amounts of snow, ice, and meltwater narrows our training

drink, then run again. Before doing so, I noted runners nearby. Once back to pace, I timed them passing a pole or other landmark ahead of me to see how much they gained, and it was almost always 7 seconds. Well before the next aid station, I caught and passed them and attached myself to another group of runners further ahead going into another aid station. Seven more seconds lost, although I kept catching and passing those whose seemingly faster tactic was to grab and run.

Given that there were eight aid stations (one every 5 kilometers) at the marathon in New Zealand, I figured I lost less than a minute by walking to drink. It's impossible to gauge how much faster I ran by being well-hydrated on a hot day, but comparing the times of my rivals to their previous bests, they seemed to lose 5 minutes. My time of 2:29:27 was faster than my recent bests, second fastest in my career at age 49.

Several years later, my son Kevin proved you could walk through aid stations and run faster still. Doing so, he ran 2:18:52 in the Lake County Marathon near Chicago to qualify for the 1984 Olympic trials. I now advise runners to practice drinking techniques during long training runs. The same techniques don't work for everybody. Find out what works for you.

options. I saw this more as a plus than a minus, in that it forced me to slow my pace and run long and slow rather than short and fast. Or I would cross-country ski. Sometimes we need breaks from the grind of continuous, hard training. In February, I ran the Cowtown Marathon in Fort Worth, Texas, and did 2:37:31, good enough for fifth overall on a windy day.

Once the snows melted in spring, I resumed my trail workouts, though I continued long runs on the roads. Despite warming weather, I stayed away from the track, but began to run twice daily to nudge my weekly mileage up closer to 100. The final week of March, I ran 99.5 miles, comfortable with my decision not to jog an extra half-mile to hit double digits. In April, I ran 2:42:05 in the Boston Marathon on a day when temperatures reached into the 70s. My best performances in May were at the Old Kent River Bank Run

SLOW VS. FAST RUNNING

It often takes years to acquire wisdom. If there is a single mistake that many distance runners make in their training, it is running too fast—particularly in long runs. In coaching marathoners, I usually recommend that they do their long runs 45 to 90 seconds slower than the pace they expect to run in the marathon. As a younger runner, I often ran my long runs at a 6:00 pace, which sounds like a mistake, but I averaged 5:30 miles in my fastest marathon. Even so, I probably trained too hard. Do what I say; not what I did!

Many marathoners worry how I can expect them to hit race pace for 26 miles if they don't run that fast in practice. (I also don't recommend runs longer than 20 miles for anybody but the most experienced runners.) The answer is that if you do run anywhere near 26 miles at or near race pace in practice, you may never make it to the race because you're injured, or you will run poorly because you are overtrained.

You accomplish many things by running your long runs at a slow pace. First, you teach your body to burn fats more efficiently, sparing glycogen so this more-efficient fuel will be available in the closing miles. Second, by running 20 miles slower than race pace, you at least approach the length of time you will run in a marathon. Third, you don't turn each workout into a race, which can be debilitating, physically and psychologically. Save your energy for speedwork, pace runs, and other fast training in the middle of the week. You can't train hard midweek if you're still recovering from a too-hard run on the weekend.

Running slow particularly makes sense for first-timers, since they don't know their marathon pace, having never run one before. Experienced runners can experiment with more miles and faster paces, because if they make a training error and either overtrain or get injured, it's not the end of the world for them. There's always another race, as I discovered during my long career as a master.

(mentioned earlier) and a 10.5-mile race on a hilly, partly gravel course in Crown Point, Indiana, where I ran 57:12 and placed first overall, shocking some good local runners, who were 20 or more years younger

> I saw bad weather more as a plus than a minus, in that it forced me to slow my pace and run long and slow rather than short and fast. Sometimes we need breaks from the grind of continuous, hard training.

than I. In June, I ran the Manitoba Marathon in Winnipeg, winning my age group in 2:32:42.

Warm weather brought a shift in training focus from distance to speed. Several days a week, I would run to a nearby golf course at sunrise and stride 10 × 100 meters, walking between. Stride, not sprint! In July, I competed in the National Masters Championships in Philadelphia, running 1500 meters in 4:22.1, not my best, but I had run the Peachtree Road Race 2 days before.

Finishing in front of me in the M45 age group in Philadelphia was Barry Almond, a running rival from several decades earlier. An Australian Olympian, Barry stayed in the United States after attending the University of Houston on a scholarship. Following my defeat, I started doing some interval training on the track, beginning with 6 × 400 and a 400 jog between. In my first workout using this pattern I averaged 69.6 quarters. Some weeks, I ran interval 200s. I still retained some of the speed from my youth, running 30-second splits. While doing speedwork, I let my weekly mileage drop into the 40- to 50-mile range.

Visiting Norway at the end of the summer, I ran 10 × 400 on the famous Bisslet Stadium track. This climaxed my interval training, and in the autumn I began to do more of my workouts in the woods with long runs on the roads. Now doing double workouts, my weekly mileage began to edge up near 80. In October, I set an M45 record of 1:06:05 for 20-K. And I placed 16th overall in "about" 2:50 at the Athens Marathon on a course that seemed several kilometers long, judging from my splits. The last week in October, I recorded 100 for the number of miles run that week. For the next several months I would be consistently near that number. In Hawaii in December for the Honolulu Marathon, I caught food poisoning and had to drop out at 8 miles. In retrospect, this may have been the best thing that could have happened to me with the championships in Christchurch only a month away, since I had a habit of racing more often than was good for me. My December mileage was actually down from the several months before.

Was I racing too often? Yes, but many of my races were tied to paid appearances where I lectured to runners. It seemed wasteful to travel to a race and not run it. Besides, those who brought me to their races naturally expected me to run.

HEADING TO NEW ZEALAND

On Sunday, January 4, I flew to New Zealand, stopping briefly in Los Angeles to run 8 miles along the oceanfront with Ron Lawrence, president of the American Medical Joggers Association. Landing in Auckland, I ran another half-dozen miles before catching the plane to Christchurch on the South Island. Although my main goal had been to compete well in the marathon, I ran 10,000 meters on the track on Thursday, placing third with 32:38 in a race won by J. K. Macdonald of New Zealand.

Running 10,000 was not unreasonable. Frank Shorter had placed fifth in that event in the 1972 Olympic Games 5 days before his marathon victory. But the following day, I did something that 2 decades later I still don't understand. Friday, I ran the 3000-meter steeplechase. It was my first 'chase in 2 years, and I never did find a rhythm, either over the hurdles or water barrier. I placed fourth in a mediocre 10:13.

During the 4 days between my last track race and the marathon, I did little running. Saturday, I ran back and forth while spectating at the cross-country events. Sunday, I did a half-dozen miles in a park and found that my legs felt recovered. Monday, I did not

> I have a habit of racing more often than is good for me.

run. Tuesday, I jogged an easy mile on grass. The marathon was on Wednesday. The weather was reasonably good: clear skies, temperatures in the mid-60s, although with some wind.

This being an international race, the course was marked in kilometers, not miles. I actually prefer kilometers to miles, since you encounter them more frequently. Particularly in the last 10 kilometers or 6 miles, the kilometers come back to you a lot faster. In a course marked in miles, it's a long way between mile 24 and mile 25.

At Christchurch, I planned to run 3:30 per kilometer, which would have given me a finishing time in the mid-2:27s. I started slowly, although keeping my eyes on Macdonald and Jeff Julian, both in my M45 age group. Julian had been one of New Zealand's top road runners 2 decades earlier. A large pack surged out ahead of us, although most of them were in the M40 division. Passing 10-K in 34:30, I learned from Jim O'Neil, a friend from California, that there was another M45 runner a minute in front of me: Eric Hunter from New Zealand.

I had been rooming with another American, Ed Rydequist, and had asked him to provide me with defizzed Coke at several points along the course. Long before Gatorade and other sports replacement drinks had become available in races around the world, I used to depend on either Coca-Cola or Pepsi-Cola to provide a boost along the way. There were two main reasons: (1) You could find Coke or Pepsi almost anywhere, and (2) you knew what you were putting into your stomach. Technically, it was against the rules to receive support away from the aid tables, and when I saw him at 15-K, Ed said he was nervous about officials nearby. He worried that he might cause my disqualification. "Just give me the Coke," I told him. "I'll take the risk."

Each time I drank, I would lose ground on those around me. This allowed Macdonald and Julian to open a 30-meter gap at 15-K. I had been using them as a shield against the wind at that point, and I suspect they pushed the pace to drop me. I struggled for a while to stay near, but their pace slowed and I caught them again by 20-K, passed in 1:09:52. By now we had caught Hunter. Eric Paulen of Australia and Fritz Mueller of the USA, both M40 runners who also were in our group, along with Piet Van Alphen of the Netherlands. Incredibly, Van Alphen was M50, holder of that age group's world record. With four from M45 running together, this was the battle for the gold medal, but I needed to keep reminding myself: not to race, not to race, not to race! It was still too early.

After the half-marathon, passed in 1:13:30, we had the wind at our backs. I pushed to stay with Paulen, Mueller, and Van Alphen, and it was around this point that the other M45 runners began to lose contact. My pack passed 30-K in 1:44:22, my split for that 10-K 34:30, equal to my time for the first 10-K, faster than the second. I held near my three companions until 33-K before yielding ground. By 38-K I had begun to struggle, but friends shouted from beside the course that I had a 1-minute lead, then 1:25 over Hunter, the next M45 runner. The next comments are from my diary, written after I had returned home.

> *I figured that unless I came completely apart I had it won. My legs were tight, and I hurt, but I continued to push, then as I got within sight of the stadium, and having looked over my shoulder to see nobody even near me, I got fired up because I had won. Most of the last kilometer I was babbling to myself, "You did it," and laughing and giving fired-up signs to nobody in particular. Coming into the stadium, I mounted a sprint down the last 50 meters of the track and leaped across the line, then continued to stagger over to the back straightaway so I could cry and talk to myself without anybody realizing what a complete idiot I was. I was happy not only because I was first in M45 and won the gold medal, my third in world competition, but also because I had broken 2:30, running 2:29:27, which made it even sweeter.*

I placed 10th overall. R. De Palmas of Italy was the M40 winner in 2:19:34. Van Alphen (1st M50) and Mueller tied for eighth in 2:27:53. Hunter placed 11th (2nd M45) in 2:30:51, with Macdonald 14th (3rd M45) in 2:32:18. Ironically, had I been 5 months older, I would have placed second to Van Alphen in the M50 marathon, but would have won gold medals in my two track races!

Except for an easy run several days later, those were my last running steps for nearly 8 weeks. I figured that after all

> I kept reminding myself: not to race, not to race, not to race! It was still too early.

those double workouts and 100-mile weeks, I needed a rest both physically and psychologically. My next diary entry was March 11, 1981, when I was tested at the Ball State University Human Performance Laboratory. David L. Costill, Ph.D., discovered significant deterioration in my fitness as measured on a treadmill. I also had gained 10 pounds: 148 versus 138 just before I left for New Zealand.

After several months of gradually tougher training, I regained most of my fitness—but not all of it. Even in June after I moved into the new age group, I was not motivated to chase records or acquire more victories. In the next 3 years, I ran 2:45 and 2:56 marathons, both times at Honolulu, but I haven't seen the bottom side of 3 hours since. No matter. I had my gold medal in the marathon, and that seemed more than enough.

LESSONS LEARNED TRAINING FOR NEW ZEALAND

1. **Planning is essential.** Success rarely comes by accident. I carefully thought out my training program a full 18 months in advance.

2. **Be smart rather than sorry.** Once your training plan is in place, don't be afraid to modify it. You can't always predict day-to-day events, including injuries. But don't get too far off track, otherwise why follow a program?

3. **Learn from previous failures.** What went wrong before? If you don't learn from your errors, you are doomed to repeat them.

4. **Determine the keys to success.** In my case it was high mileage. As a 4:13 miler, I knew I had the speed. I also knew

I had to crank my miles up to survive the marathon's final miles. I ran numerous 20-milers and peaked over 100 weekly miles to improve endurance.

5. **Prepare for all eventualities.** Knowing the marathon would be held in New Zealand's summer, I devised a drinking strategy of walking through aid stations to maximize fluid intake. I practiced this strategy in earlier races.

6. **Seek support.** To ensure ample fluids, and the right fluids, I recruited a friend to hand me containers of de-fizzed Coke at precise points along the course.

7. **Don't panic.** Even though I watched my main rivals pull away from me in the first miles, I didn't chase them, figuring that if I held my pace I would see them later. I did.

8. **Avoid diversions.** In hindsight, I made the mistake of racing too often, even during the "taper period" leading into the marathon. I ran two other track races at the championships, which probably was not wise, even though I got away with doing it.

9. **Include postrace rest.** I knew once the marathon was past and the 18-month effort done, I was going to rest myself both mentally and physically. I went 2 months afterward when I barely ran a step—although I did do some cross-country skiing.

10. **Savor the victory.** Championships and records lost their appeal for me after this final marathon victory. Ten years later, I cranked my training up another notch and won my fourth gold medal at the Worlds in the steeplechase. That probably is enough gold for my career.

7 ALTERNATIVES

For Masters, Multiple Sports Provide a Means to an End

Despite my 2-month running hiatus during the winter of 1981, I did not remain entirely inactive. I did some skiing, both downhill and cross-country. I lifted weights, aware that during high-mileage training—such as the lead-up to a marathon—I often overlook upper-body strength. After the snow melted, I started biking. When the water in the lake warmed, I added swimming. By then, I was back running, working out on the track, pounding the trails in the woods again, and participating in at least a few road races.

Most runners today would label such activity cross-training, although I did not think of it as such. I was simply having fun, spinning my wheels figuratively and literally, while deciding which goal to select next. If the term cross-training had been invented by the year 1981, it certainly had not penetrated the public consciousness, nor mine.

Several decades before, as an arrogant submaster, I knew the only activity that would make me a better runner was running: twice a day, 100 miles a week. That makes sense if you're in your twenties, trying to qualify for an Olympic team or win the Boston Marathon. It may not make sense if you're in your forties, participating in much lower-profile masters sports. It definitely does not make sense once

you move into your six-
ties, where your most
important goal may be
staying alive.

> A lesson that most masters runners need to learn is that less is often best.

One truth on which
most exercise scientists agree is that if you want to succeed in any
sport, and particularly in running, you need to practice that sport
almost to the exclusion of any other activity. David L. Costill, Ph.D.,
founder of the Ball State University Human Performance Laboratory, states it clearly: "Training is usually sports-specific. You don't
spend 2 hours daily in a pool if you want to achieve success as a
runner. And champion swimmers would be wasting their time running quarters on a track or going for 20-mile bike rides."

The Kenyans don't cross-train. The Ethiopians don't cross-train.
Most of them don't own a fast bike, and if you threw them into a
pool, they would sink quickly to the bottom, having so little body
fat. They succeed by running, running, running: two, sometimes
three times a day. If you suggested cross-training to the Kenyans,
they would be too polite to laugh, but after you got out of sight, they
would roll their eyes and smile at each other.

Nevertheless, there are exceptions to the rule of sports specificity,
as Dr. Costill would be quick to acknowledge. A runner might spend
those several hours daily in a pool if injured and unable to run.
Megan Leahy, a girl I coached in high school, did just that. I supervised Megan's running her first 2 years at Elston High School in
Michigan City, Indiana. Another coach took charge her junior and
senior years. He trained her and her teammates much harder than I
dared, raising them to the level where they won two state cross-
country championships, but Megan also suffered a series of injuries.
She missed nearly the entire dual meet season in cross-country her
senior year. Megan trained daily in the pool and healed enough to
start running again just before the qualifying rounds leading to the
state meet. She placed first in the sectionals, first in the regionals,
first in the semistate, and second in the state championships.

It is tempting to suggest that Megan might have won the state title
if able to focus her attention on running, but in truth, she might have

overtrained and done worse. That is a lesson that most masters runners need to learn: Less is often best. Slender, possessed of a fragile body, a doe instead of a deer, Megan spent most of her college career at Indiana University battling one injury after another, running well, but not quite up to her level of accomplishment as a high schooler. After graduating from Indiana, Megan enrolled in podiatry school. "I've had every running injury imaginable," she told me. "Maybe I can help prevent injuries in others."

Cross-training will enable you to maintain, if not build, strength and aerobic fitness while recovering from injury. That is one exception to the rule of sports specificity. The other exception is that as we age as runners, it becomes increasingly more difficult to maintain a regimen of running daily—and forget twice daily. Masters runners might be lucky to get two good running workouts a week.

A SHOCKING SPORT

Running is a contact sport. Unlike sports such as football, hockey, basketball, and baseball, we don't collide with our opponents; we collide with the pavement. Our feet hit the ground as often as a hundred times a minute, shocking our musculoskeletal systems with foot impacts several times our body weight. Not all of us possess perfect biomechanics, so as we run, our feet, ankles, knees, hips, and associated muscles and ligaments twist to keep us in balance. If, like me, you had seen slow-motion studies of the lower limbs twisting during each foot strike, you would wonder how we can run at all. Orthotics and well-designed shoes can help dissipate some of the ground-contact shock, and correct some of the twisting, but not all of it. Muscles also tear and repair after we run long or fast, part of the system that eventually will make us stronger and faster. Particularly after a hard workout of interval quarters on the track or a tempo run in the woods, our bodies need a day or two or three or more to recover before we can train hard again.

This is true of young athletes, too. One of the greatest middle-distance runners of all time was Great Britain's Sebastian Coe, setter of multiple world records from 800 through 2000 meters, two-time

JUMP IN THE POOL

The single best alternative to running—if you have a lower body injury—is aquarunning: using a flotation vest in deep water and mimicking the running movements as closely as possible. You need to own or borrow a vest and you need a pool deep enough so you can make the movements without touching bottom, but training this way is simple and effective.

If uninjured, however, it's easier just to swim. Any stroke: crawl, back, breast, even treading water. There are two periods during the year when I swim as a form of cross-training. In the winter in Ponte Vedra Beach, Florida, I swim in a heated outdoor pool at The Lodge and Club's fitness center, only 1 minute's walk from our condo. In the summer, I swim in Lake Michigan across the street from our home in Long Beach, Indiana. Important in my choice of this cross-training exercise is convenience.

This leaves a gap of several months between: both spring and fall, when I do no swimming, because the lake's too cold. Rather than take 15 minutes to drive to the YMCA, I use other forms of cross-training. In Florida, the Atlantic Ocean is only another minute's walk away from our condo, but I rarely swim there. I don't like swimming in rough water either in the ocean or the lake. People drown every summer in the lake near our home because they don't recognize the danger from riptides that may carry them out over their heads in a matter of seconds.

I also run in the water in both places. In the lake, I run in chest-deep water parallel to shore. The lake has a soft and sandy bottom, so I don't even

Olympic gold medalist in the 1500, two-time silver medalist in the 800. A month before Seb ran a 1500 and 800 gold-silver double at the 1984 Olympic Games in Los Angeles, I observed him training at the York High School track west of Chicago. He ran a classic interval workout of 20 × 200 meters with a circling jog of maybe 25 to 45 seconds between sprints, averaging 27 seconds for each repeat. He ran the final 200 in a stunning 22.5 seconds, fast enough to win most high-school races at that distance. I could hardly believe the numbers I saw on my digital watch.

need aquashoes. I do use a wet suit vest for buoyancy as much as for warmth. Typically, I swim in one direction anywhere from 200 to 800 meters, then turn and run back. It takes a lot longer to run a specific distance in the water than on shore, so this provides a good workout. Time thus becomes a more important factor than distance in dictating how much I do. This is true when I bike or swim as well. I consider running in the lake a pleasant diversion, particularly on a sunny day, and hardly think of it as cross-training.

The Florida pool is for lap-swimming and aerobics classes, so it has no deep end. After a half-hour in the weight room, I swim laps for 10 to 20 minutes, then finish with 5 to 10 minutes of running. That's a good hour of training. I exaggerate my running movements in the water to promote both strength and flexibility. Running in the water thus becomes a form of dynamic stretching. In Florida, where I can measure myself against swimmers in other lanes, I'm usually the slowest. That doesn't bother me. I don't do kick turns, and I usually pause for 5 to 10 seconds at each end before pushing off. I'm in the pool to burn a few calories and strengthen my upper body, not to train for a triathlon. (When in triathlon training, I used to swim much farther.)

While I've been swimming in the lake for several decades, I only started lap-swimming recently. I thought doing repetitive laps would be horribly boring with nothing to look at but the bottom of the pool, but surprised myself by finding my water workouts rather soothing.

After the workout, Sebastian Coe and I talked for an article I was writing for *The Runner* magazine. Seb admitted that when he was younger, he could do workouts of that intensity 4 and 5 days in a row. "Now that I'm older," he said, "I realize that I need more rest between hard workouts if I hope to avoid injury." At that time, Sebastian Coe was 27 years old!

That is a lesson we must learn and—most important—must apply as masters runners. We do need more rest. We need to train with some intensity, but we need to moderate that intensity. And we also need to determine which cross-training exercises work best for us in preserving, if not building, fitness if we want to avoid injury and perform at peak potential.

While working on this book, I participated in a research study designed by Mark Sleeper, an exercise scientist and physical therapy instructor at Northwestern University School of Medicine in Chicago. Sleeper was testing older people, both runners and non-runners, to see if the former had better balance, meaning we would be less likely to fall and injure ourselves.

Yes, we are less at risk, he eventually discovered. But while I was having wires and sensing devices connected to my body so I could stand on a force plate and be knocked off balance while being filmed by a half-dozen cameras, Sleeper and I chatted. I mentioned a comment by Larry Mengelkoch, Ph.D., quoted earlier in this book that at least in our forties and fifties, if we can maintain the same volume and intensity of training as in our twenties and thirties, we can continue to perform at nearly the same level. Our performance curve may slant downward, but not that much. That was the prime message in the 20-year longitudinal study Michael L. Pollock, Ph.D., had done with two dozen elite masters competitors, a study in which Dr. Mengelkoch had assisted.

Now, the conundrum: As we age, for various reasons, it becomes increasingly difficult to maintain the same volume and intensity in our training. I managed it through my forties, but not through my fifties. If, as masters, we run the same number of miles, we find ourselves forced to run them more slowly. If we run at the same pace, we find ourselves unable to run as many miles. Thus the conundrum and chicken-before-egg question: Do our volume and intensity drop because we age, or do we age because our volume and intensity drop?

Sleeper conceded the point based on his own experience as a runner and that of his wife, Debbie. They were both in their forties. She had started running competitively at age 12, averaging 2,500 miles a year through age 30. Her fastest 10-K time was sub-40:00; the fastest of her seven marathons, 3:35. As she moved into her forties, Debbie found it difficult to find the time to train as much, plus she had begun to experience hip problems. Her mileage dropped to less than 1,000 miles a year. Her 10-K times are now over 45:00; her marathon times over 4 hours. A track runner of medium ability in high school and college, Mark Sleeper found that he too no longer could run as far or as fast as he liked, both in training and in races. His 13-year-old daughter, principally a gymnast, recently had run 1600 meters (just under a mile) in less than 6 minutes. He was both sad and delighted that she now was faster than he was.

"It's a matter of impact," Sleeper suggested. "Over the years, all the impact we experience running adds up and takes a toll on our systems. For a while, our muscles and ligaments absorb the punishment and dissipate the forces, but eventually we begin to wear out. If we want to continue to maintain a high level of fitness, we need to change our training." Commuting from the western suburbs, Sleeper now rides his bike 4 miles to the train station many mornings and 4 miles back in the evenings.

For him and for many masters runners, cross-training is a matter of survival.

TAKE IT TO THE SLOPES

My first encounter with cross-training came the winter of my senior year at Carleton College in Northfield, Minnesota. Following my conversations with better-trained runners on the infield grass at the 1952 NCAA Track and Field Championships in Berkeley, California, I committed myself to becoming a full-time runner. That's not easy in Minnesota where minus-zero temperatures are common, and where snow and ice on the roads can make running difficult if not impossible. Winter can grind you down in the upper Midwest, robbing you of your motivation to run outdoors, particularly in your first year as a full-time runner.

As masters, we need to determine which cross-training exercises work best for us in preserving, if not building, fitness if we want to avoid injury and perform at peak potential.

I split my time that

winter between running and cross-country skiing. Carleton had no professor to coach the ski team at that time. In charge of the squad was John McCamant, a sophomore and teammate of mine in cross-country and track. John had placed in the top 10 that fall in cross-country and would win the 880 in a time of 1:55 later that spring in track. Between those seasons, he skied.

At John's urging, I joined with the ski team several times for cross-country ski workouts. To compete in ski meets back then, you needed to participate in all four events, which included, in addition to cross-country skiing, ski jumping and downhill and slalom racing, events for which I had neither the skills nor the interest. But skiing on the same Arboretum trails that I ran during the fall turned out to be fun, despite inadequate equipment. Downhill skis in that era were narrower than today's wide models, almost like today's Telemark skis. Downhill skiers wore leather boots. The boots attached to the skis with cable bindings that fit through two clips on each side of the ski, anchoring heels and skis, making turning easier. To ski cross-country, you simply unhitched the cable from the clips, allowing your heels to rise on each stride. In all honesty, because of the slow and inadequate equipment, cross-country skiing back then was not a lot of fun.

As I improved as a runner in the next several years, I abandoned skiing, particularly downhill skiing. A bad fall on a black-diamond slope at Aspen, Colorado, resulted in a twisted knee that still bothers me 50 years later. That convinced me that skiing was too dangerous for someone intent on Olympic success. Several decades passed, and my concept of what was important in life changed. I was 48 years old when one of my neighbors, Alf Djubik, a Norwegian, suggested I give Nordic (cross-country) skiing a try. By then, cross-country and downhill equipment had evolved in separate directions. Nordic skis were longer, narrower, and lighter. Boots resembled running shoes. Suddenly, the sport was fun. I found that skiing my regular running trails took the edge off winter.

> Running is a contact sport. Unlike sports such as football, we don't collide with our opponents; we collide with the pavement.

More than that, I embraced cross-country skiing as a competitive sport, training for it with the same seriousness I applied to running. I competed regularly in races, including the American Birkebeiner, a 51-K ski race over a hilly trail between Telemark Lodge and Hayward, Wisconsin. Ironically, Telemark Lodge was the same resort where I had skied during semester breaks my first 3 years at Carleton. With the advent of jet travel and quick flights to Colorado, few downhill skiers visited Telemark any more, so owner Tony Wise converted the lodge into a cross-country mecca, the "Birkie," attracting 6,000 or more competitors each year.

Cross-country skiing, I quickly realized, was the perfect winter cross training complement to my running. It was a total fitness exercise. The fact that I cross-country skied, I later reasoned, was one reason why I scored so well in Mike Pollock's longitudinal study of aging masters athletes. In terms of aerobic fitness, no exercise comes close to matching cross-country skiing. My peak maximum VO_2 was 72, approximately the same as Olympic marathon champion Frank Shorter. (Frank was lighter and faster and more efficient biomechanically, explaining the 11-minute difference in our marathon times.) A few elite runners have been tested with maximum VO_2 scores in the 80s. Such scores are routine among elite cross-country skiers, including Juha Mieto, an Olympic gold medalist from Finland. I encountered Mieto one year at a Nordic ski race at Holmenkollen outside Oslo. He stood nearly a foot taller than I and had shoulders like a linebacker. No way could Mieto succeed as a runner, but he was perfectly configured for the sport in which he excelled.

With the possible exception of aquarunning (using a flotation vest), cross-country skiing is perhaps the perfect cross-training exercise for runners. You don't merely maintain your cardiovascular fitness; you can build it along with your upper body. Not only do you exercise the muscles of your lower body, but the aggressive poling exercises the much-neglected muscles of the upper body. Skis slide through the snow, so there is next to no impact. There are two basic techniques used in Nordic ski races. The "classic" technique involves straight-ahead movements in precisely set twin tracks.

EMBRACE WINTER

Too many runners new to the sport abandon running once temperatures drop below freezing and snow starts to fly. They either head indoors to run on treadmills in comfortably heated fitness centers, or they don't run at all.

To maintain and maximize your running ability, you need to embrace winter. You'll enjoy the cold months more if you banish negative thoughts and become involved in outdoor sports such as snowshoeing and cross-country skiing. As long as you dress warmly, there's no reason you can't continue to run outdoors as well. Here are the activities that work best.

Outdoor running. Don't worry about running fast. Just cover the distance at a comfortable pace. Consider the extra weight of winter clothes as a form of resistance training.

Indoor running. Most fitness centers offer multiple treadmills for their members. Or buy one for your basement gym, although the best 'mills are not cheap.

Snowshoeing. Easy to learn, plus you can wear your regular running clothes and shoes. When the snow is too icy or too thin to run on, or even too deep, you can still snowshoe on it.

Cross-country skiing. A total-body workout that strengthens shoulders and arms. There are two cross-country techniques: skating and classic. Classic is best for runners, because it uses straight-ahead movements.

Aquarunning. Running or swimming in a pool offers another winter option. Best is using a flotation vest, but you also can run in shallow water or swim using various strokes.

Stationary bicycling. Indoor biking is a good quad-strengthening workout.

Faster is the skating technique that involves sideways movements on packed snow, the movements similar to those used by inline skaters. The classic (and somewhat slower) technique probably works best for cross-training runners, because the straight-ahead movements utilize the muscles similarly to the way they are used in running. Nevertheless, if you want to become a cross-country skier, pick whichever technique you enjoy most—or use both.

Week	Sun	Mon	Tue	Wed	Thu	Fri	Sat
1	Ski 30–60 min	Swim & strength	Run 30 min	Bike & strength	Run 30 min	Rest	Run 30–60 min
2	Snow-shoe 30 60 min	Run 30 min	Swim & strength	Run 30 min	Bike & strength	Rest	Ski 30–60 min

It's tougher than biking outdoors, since you can't coast down hills.

Strength training. An indoor activity that you should do year-round anyway.

For an effective training schedule, run 2 or 3 days a week. With snow on the ground, add or substitute 2 or 3 days of cross-country skiing or snow-shoeing. Blend in other cross-training activities to suit your needs and interest. For example, a gym workout could include strength training, bicycling, and swimming. Once spring arrives, you can shift your focus back to running as your principle sport. Here's a 2-week winter cross-training program that would benefit all masters runners.

With a little experience, you can design your own winter training schedule. Weather conditions may dictate whether you can run or ski or snowshoe outdoors, so be flexible scheduling activities. Don't sit still too long, and spring will soon be near.

One downside about skiing that scares many runners away is that it is a very technical sport demanding specific skills. Plus it can be dangerous, particularly if you downhill ski or snowboard. Yes, there is impact if you slide off the trail and into a tree. Also, I discovered that cross-country skiing so developed my cardiovascular system that I could become injured if I made too sudden a switch back to running. This happened one year when I spent several weeks skiing in Norway, then headed south to Italy where I ran several road races. The too-quick switch was like putting a Porsche engine in a Volkswagen chassis. My fine-tuned cardiovascular system pushed me to run at a pace faster than my running muscles could tolerate. The lesson learned was to blend running with skiing throughout the winter. I often did this by running with skis and poles a half-mile to the golf course near my home and, after an hour or so of skiing, running back. Otherwise, if there was snow on the ground, I skied; if the roads were clear, I ran.

Some years later, I discovered snowshoeing as an equally good cross-training alternative for winter. In many respects, snowshoeing is better than skiing, because you can actually run on snowshoes, not as fast as on the road, but with similar motions. I obtained a pair of snowshoes from Barney Klecker, a 2:15 marathoner, who once set a world 50-mile record of 4:51:25. For several years, Barney manu-

SNOWSHOEING

More and more runners have begun to discover snowshoeing as a form of optional winter training. Consequently, manufacturers now offer snowshoes designed for running in snow as opposed to crossing deep drifts. Snowshoe races have begun to attract runners and cross-country skiers in the northern states. Many of the better ski stores now carry snowshoes, but if you're a masters runner, make sure that you purchase narrow snowshoes suitable for moving fast. If the salesperson doesn't know what you're talking about, find another salesperson or another store.

During a visit to Crested Butte in Colorado, my wife, Rose, and I signed up for a snowshoe tour with three of our grandchildren: Kyle, Wesley, and Angela. Renting snowshoes, we rode the lift up to the top of one of the downhill runs, then followed a trail that wound through the woods back to the base. Winter Park is another Colorado resort that offers guided snowshoe tours. We snowshoed there several years earlier. After we got off the lift, we disappeared into the woods and, despite the presence of lifts and downhill slopes nearby, we might have been miles from civilization. Snow-

factured and sold snowshoes as a part-time sideline to his teaching. Barney's wife was Janis Klecker, who won the 1992 Olympic marathon trial in 2:30:12. The race was held in Houston in January, and Janis spent most of the previous several months alternating between running on the roads and running in the snow with snowshoes. Unlike cross-country skiing, which sometimes takes years to master, the learning curve with snowshoes is almost instantaneous. One time while injured in the summer, Janis ran in snowshoes on a golf course to reduce impact during her recovery. This raised numerous eyebrows among those who saw her, but it speeded Janis's return to running.

TRIPLE THREAT

About the same time I rediscovered skiing as an alternate winter sport, I also discovered an alternative summer sport in the triathlon,

---

shoeing provides a unique experience for ski resort guests who prefer to avoid or limit the downhill experience.

Once you get the snowshoes on your feet, you'll be surprised how easy it is to walk or run on them. The learning curve for a fit person is about 30 seconds. Just start walking or running. No expensive lessons necessary. You can wear boots, but I just wear my regular running shoes, or sometimes mukluks. The best running shoes to use are those designed for running on trails, since they usually offer more protection, including a tight fit around the ankle so snow can't get in. You may bang your ankles until you get used to the movements. If so, use ankle pads similar to those used for soccer.

Perhaps the greatest advantage of snowshoeing is that it allows you access into parts of the woods that you might not otherwise be able to penetrate. At the Indiana Dunes State Park near Chesterton, Indiana, if you wander much more than 50 meters off the marked trails in the summer, you can easily become disoriented and lost. But if lost on snowshoes, you simply retrace your tracks.

Plus snowshoeing is a lot of fun.

an event that combines swimming, cycling, and running. The world's oldest and best-known three-event race is the

> Like Alice in Wonderland, I had to run fast just to keep up.

Ironman Triathlon, founded in February 1978 by John Collins, a naval commander stationed in Hawaii, who got in an argument with some friends at a local running race over who were the best athletes: swimmers, cyclists, or runners. To settle a bet, Collins suggested an event that combined the course of the Waikiki Rough Water Swim (2.4 miles), a bike ride around the island of Oahu (112 miles), and the Honolulu Marathon (26.2 miles). "The winner," Collins declared, "will be called an ironman."

Only 15 competitors appeared that first year, but ABC began televising the Ironman Triathlon in 1980, sparking additional interest. John Wilson, a member of the Dunes Running Club in northwestern Indiana, suggested that we conduct a similar race, but with shorter distances. Club members designed a course at LaLumiere High School that began with a pond swim that couldn't have been much more than 100 meters around a buoy. We next jumped on our bikes and pedaled a hilly 8 miles around the countryside before finishing on the high school's cross-country course, which added several more miles. It was fun and easily accessible to anyone in reasonably good shape, and we repeated the race the following year before moving it to a better-designed course in the city of LaPorte. In only its fourth year, the LaPorte Triathlon attracted 450 competitors and was one of the largest triathlons in the United States. The event continues to attract near that number, although other triathlons now are much bigger.

Most early years I won my age group, because the swim was short, as was the biking leg, and if anyone with more ability in those sports got out in front of me, I usually was fast enough to run them down on the last, running leg. No specific skills seemed necessary. Train for the triathlon? I usually swam and biked in the summer anyway, so why bother?

But within a few years, as the Ironman Triathlon in Hawaii grew in size and popularity, more and more triathlons appeared to challenge participants from each of the three sports. Many of these early triathletes from the start of the 1980s were the same baby boomers who had made running such a popular sport in the late 1970s. Perhaps bored with running 10-K and marathon races, they saw the addition of swimming and bicycling as the next step in their athletic careers. They began to train seriously in all three disciplines so they could compete better. They also began to upgrade their equipment.

I reluctantly went along. Although I still swam only when Lake Michigan warmed in June or July, I bought a new ten-speed bicycle and started to ride occasionally with a local group of cyclists. The cyclists moved pretty swiftly in a tight chain, but I found I could remain with them as long as I stayed tucked into their draft. I also began to combine workouts where I swam and ran, or biked and ran. Within a few years, I found myself competing in more triathlons than running races during the summer.

One triathlon I enjoyed began at Indiana Beach near the town of Monticello and finished on the Purdue University campus in West Lafayette. A fraternity and sorority organized the event as a fundraiser for charity and as an excuse to drink some beer on a sunny Saturday afternoon. We began with a mile swim in Lake Shafer, formed behind a dam in the Tippecanoe River. Jumping on our bikes, we cycled 50 miles past cornfields on back country roads. The final leg was a 15-K run.

Swimming for me always was a matter of survival, but once on the bike, I usually was able to maintain a steady pace near 20 mph, which allowed me to catch and pass at least some of the faster swimmers. The first year at Purdue, another competitor came flying past me on the bicycle leg. What impressed me was not how good a cyclist he was, but how bad he must have been as a swimmer to come out of the water behind me. I don't know if I caught him on the final leg running, but I passed a lot of other competitors, and nobody passed me. Two weeks before the triathlon, I had run a 15-K at the Blueberry Stomp in Plymouth, Indiana, winning my age group in about 54 minutes. My Purdue time over the same distance was 56 minutes, only 2 minutes slower.

I returned to West Lafayette 2 years later, not much improved as a swimmer, but definitely a swifter cyclist, the result of more serious training in that sport plus the addition of special pedals that locked my shoes in place, permitting faster speeds because I could both push and pull on each revolution. I cut 15 minutes off my cycling time. Unfortunately, in focusing on that triathlon discipline, I developed too-strong quads, so my running efficiency declined. It was partly a matter of poor pacing; I had become so focused on learning to cycle better, I forgot what I did best: run. Like Alice in Wonderland, I had to run fast just to keep up.

The sport was changing around me. I appeared one year at the Muncie Endurathon, a triathlon with half-ironman distances.

TRI-FIT

If you are interested in general fitness, no better combination of exercises exists than the three events of the triathlon: swimming, cycling, and running. Swimming develops the upper-body muscles. Cycling and running develop the lower-body muscles, although somewhat different ones. (Cycling's focus is more on the quadriceps; running, the hamstrings and calves.) All three exercises develop the cardiovascular system, running probably the best of the three. Add an occasional walk as a respite from running; strength train a couple of days weekly; stretch when the opportunity presents itself; and you come pretty close to possessing the total fitness that will allow you to live both longer and better.

The theory behind using triathlon events for fitness is that if you push your running muscles hard one day, you can rest them by swimming or biking the next day. Be cautious, however. By shifting from stressed muscles to rested muscles, you can train too hard on days when easy workouts are prescribed. This opens the door to injuries and overtraining.

Here is a 4-week tri-fit schedule for those whose goal is physical fitness as much as running a fast 5-K. The schedule suggests three running workouts a week. If your main competitive focus is running, you probably will want to make those your hard workouts. I have prescribed time rather than

Checking in at the bicycle inspection, I noticed that while I had upgraded my bike with locking pedals, almost everybody else now had special handle-

> I respect competitors in the triathlon, but unlike running, it's a sport where you can buy faster times.

bars that permitted a lower and more aerodynamic position. The next purchase for $500 would be a solid rear wheel, also faster, and if you wanted to nibble a few more minutes and seconds off your bike leg time, you could spend $2,000 for a titanium bike. Almost every other competitor at Muncie that year sported a wet suit, not for warmth since the temperature of the lake was near 80 degrees, but

Week	Sun	Mon	Tue	Wed	Thu	Fri	Sat
1	Walk 60 min	Bike & strength	Run 30 min	Strength & swim	Run 30 min	Rest	Run 60 min
2	Bike 60 min	Run 30 min	Strength & swim	Run 30 min	Bike & strength	Rest	Walk 60 min
3	Run 60 min	Strength & swim	Run 30 min	Bike 60 min	Run & strength	Rest	Run 60 min
4	Walk 60 min	Run 30 min	Strength & swim	Run 30 min	Bike & strength	Rest	Run 60 min

distance, since people differ in ability to cover miles in each of the three sports. On several days, I suggest strength training. This is best done after your biking or running rather than before. But I like to swim after strength training rather than before. Weather conditions also may determine which days you do certain workouts.

The tri-fit schedule only suggests how you might train. Try different combinations to see what works best for you. Be flexible. And toward that end, don't forget to stretch.

for buoyancy and a faster swim time. By the time I emerged from the water, there were very few bikes other than mine in the changeover corral. I re-

> She rode a bike that looked like the one ridden by the Wicked Witch of the West in *The Wizard of Oz.*

spected competitors in the triathlon, but unlike running, it appeared to be a sport where you could buy faster times. Although I qualified for the Ironman Triathlon at Muncie, I was unwilling to commit myself to the extra training (swimming year-round) that might have allowed me to be competitive in that much longer race. I sometimes regret that decision. Within a few years, I drifted away from both cross-country skiing and the triathlon as competitive sports and returned my attention to running as my prime focus. Turning 60, I won my fourth gold medal at the World Masters Championships in Turku, Finland. Obviously, my triathlon training had not slowed me down much, plus it helped me maintain my motivation to stay physically fit.

And as I continue to age, I appreciate even more the other two triathlon disciplines as alternative exercises for masters runners. If you want to train 6 or 7 days a week, yet are unable to recover quick enough to run that often, swimming and cycling provide good options along with skiing and snowshoeing in the winter—although don't overlook walking, either.

Having upgraded my bicycle equipment so that I could be competitive in triathlons, I recently downgraded that same equipment for social reasons. My wife's bicycle of choice is a mountain bike with wide tires, a kickstand, and a basket for carrying items. I would kid her about having a bike that looked like the one ridden by the Wicked Witch of the West in *The Wizard of Oz,* but she seemed much more comfortable than I did hunched over my handlebars on my thin-tired bike, able to see little more than the asphalt pavement in front of me. Soon, I bought a mountain bike of my own, which slowed my maximum speed by 5 or 10 mph, but speed no longer motivated me.

Maybe I was getting older, but I also began to worry about the dangers of going fast on a bike. I stopped training with the group from the local bike shop after one evening when we were riding in a chain through a rural area east of Chesterton, Indiana. We came to a slight downhill that couldn't have offered much more than a 1-degree drop, but it caused one of the leaders to say, "Let's see how fast we can go." Pedaling fast downhill, I had reached 36 mph when I passed a house where a dog came charging out of the yard toward me. I visualized him colliding with my front wheel with resulting damage to both of us. Fortunately, I slid on by unharmed, but not every cyclist is lucky enough to avoid serious injury. The founder of the masters movement, David H. R. Pain, was rolling down a hill near San Diego at 41 mph when a tire blew, catapulting him over the handlebars and onto the pavement. He wound up in the hospital with several fractured ribs, a fractured scapula, a concussion, two collapsed lungs, a bruised heart, and vertigo, plus a major case of road rash. He was in intensive care for 7 days and bedridden for 4 weeks. David was 81 at the time and while seemingly having been given a warning to retire, he was back on the bike and participating in 50-mile rides within a year of his accident.

Is it a sign of age or maturity that I now achieve more enjoyment bicycling with my wife, our only goal fitness rather than trophies? Wait, I take that back. Our real goal is coffee and rolls. During the summer, we cycle 2 or 3 days a week to one of about a half-dozen coffee shops near our home in Long Beach, Indiana. All the coffeehouses we visit seem to get deliveries from the same bakery. My favorite treat is an almond roll, almonds reportedly being a nutritional plus for your health. We sit outdoors in the warm sun sipping our coffee and chatting with other coffee-shop regulars. Depending on which coffee shop we select, this means a ride of between 6 and 14 miles. The furthest coffee shop is in New Buffalo, Michigan, the same interim destination that was the focus of my 13.5-mile cross-country workouts leading up to victory in the 1972 Longest Day Marathon.

> I achieve more enjoyment bicycling with my wife, our only goal fitness rather than trophies.

Life changes. The difference between then and now is that I previously would never stop for coffee and an almond roll.

Will bicycling to a coffee shop 3 days a week improve my ability as a masters runner? Not really, but it certainly allows me to spend more time communicating with my wife, who earlier in my running career often got left behind when I rushed off to track meets and road races. While down in Florida, we also go for walks of several miles along Ponte Vedra Beach, which at low tide is perfect for walking or running. Sometimes Rose will walk while I jog on ahead, but I find that my jogging pace now is not that much faster than her walking pace. (You know you've slowed down as a masters runner when female power walkers speed on past you.) I'll run

TRI-FAST

Once you become tri-fit (page 148), consider becoming tri-fast. By increasing the amount of swimming and cycling in your training program, you can become a triathlete. For your first triathlon, pick a small, local race that you can complete in an hour or so, rather than an ironman or even half-ironman triathlon, with their ultradistances. Save that experience for later. Don't be ashamed to show up at the starting line with a bike that has a basket and kickstand.

The secret to becoming a triathlete is learning to train for several activities at the same time. It's not enough to swim, cycle, or run on different days of the week. You need to do at least a few workouts where you move from the water onto a bike or shift from biking to running. Transitions are key to triathlon success: not merely shortening the length of time it takes to change clothes, but also adapting your muscles to the changes. It's not easy to get off a bike, cramped from being unable to change position, and reach your full running stride.

As with the tri-fit program, I have prescribed times rather than distances. We all differ in our ability to absorb hard training. The following 4-week schedule will get you started and prepare you for a short-distance triathlon. Feel free to adapt the schedule to your own needs. Once you finish

for 5 minutes and look around only to find that I barely have gained 100 meters on her. The only thing that allows me

> You know you've slowed down when female power walkers speed on past you.

to maintain my lead is that she stops frequently to pick up shells and sharks' teeth.

Also in Florida, I work out 3 or 4 days a week at the fitness center that is part of The Lodge and Club, only a minute's walk across a boardwalk over a marsh from our condo. There was an alligator that lived in the marsh that we usually looked for, but after swallowing a 30-pound dog one day, he was removed to a locale farther from

your first triathlon, there are many additional training programs online and in other books (including my *How to Train*) that will teach you how to improve.

Week	Sun	Mon	Tue	Wed	Thu	Fri	Sat
1	Swim/ run 45 min	Strength	Run 30 min	Bike 45 min	Run/ strength 45 min	Rest	Run 30 min
2	Swim/ bike 50 min	Strength	Bike/ run 35 min	Bike/ strength 45 min	Swim/ run 45 min	Rest	Run 40 min
3	Swim/ run 55 min	Strength	Run 40 min	Bike 60 min	Run/ strength 45 min	Rest	Run 50 min
4	Swim/ bike 60 min	Strength	Bike/ run 45 min	Bike/ strength 60 min	Swim/ run 45 min	Rest	Run 60 min

civilization. Rose participates in an aquacise class almost daily. I use the weight room, then swim and run in the water. It's a good life.

Walking, swimming, cycling, running. Throw in some strength training. Don't forget to stretch. It is the perfect recipe for fitness and longevity. Whether it is a recipe for maintaining your ability to run fast 10-Ks and marathons is another question, but sometimes our priorities change.

Here's how to use alternative sports to become a better runner and a fitter person.

1. **Pick a cross-training activity you enjoy.** Why waste time in activities that are not fun? Cross-training runners have enough choices of alternative sports, so compatibility should be an important consideration.

2. **If injured, pick a sport similar to running.** Your focus in rehabbing probably should be maintaining your hard-earned run conditioning. Aquarunning is best if a pool is handy. Consult your doctor regarding what you can and can't do.

3. **For fitness, pick a sport different from running.** It's hard to beat the triathlon combination of swimming, bicycling, and running if your goal is total fitness.

4. **Not all sports complement your running.** This is particularly true if you are training for a marathon. As the long run mileage hits the upper double digits, sports that involve side movements, such as basketball, soccer, and tennis, can increase your risk of injury.

5. **Be certain of your focus.** I found cross-country skiing and triathlons so addictive that they hampered my running ability. That's okay for a change of pace, so it depends on what is most important to you.

6. **Strength training is important for success.** That's true in all sports. It's also true for fitness. Running is a one-dimensional sport that strengthens some muscles, but not others. Pumping iron may not make you faster, but it can make you healthier.

7. **Don't overlook stretching.** Flexibility becomes more and more important as we age. Stretching may or may not prevent injury, but it certainly can help you move better. That's the secret to looking younger than your actual age.

8. **Don't overlook simple sports.** Walking is a great cross-training exercise, but too many runners overlook its benefits. Make this your easy-day activity, as well as a way to communicate with significant others who may not share your running skills.

8 ESSENTIALS

Strength Training, Stretching, and Common Sense Make You a Better Master

In 1958, I traveled to York, Pennsylvania, for the National AAU 30-Kilometer Championships. Swift-flying jet planes and intercontinental expressways had not yet revolutionized the way we traveled. I took the train from Chicago to Philadelphia, then hitched a ride with Browning Ross, a two-time Olympian, who published a small newsletter called *Long Distance Log*. Browning's *Log* featured race results only. Monthly, with barely a dozen pages, the *Log* easily recorded the name of every finisher in every road race in the United States. With a circulation of a few hundred at most, Browning made little profit; his was a labor of love. That same year of 1958, Ross founded the Road Runners Club of America, whose grassroots approach to race organization would sow the seeds for the running boom that followed 2 decades later. By the early 1980s, *Runner's World* reached half a million readers and could publish only a fraction of the results of hundreds of road races held each year.

But in 1958, life was simpler. Only a few dozen runners appeared for the 30-K in York. The race was run on a multilap course. It was rainy, cold. In what was my first road race longer than 10 miles, I ran with leaders Bob Carman of Pittsburgh and Al Confalone of the Boston Athletic Association until the last several miles, when the two of them pulled away, Carman eventually winning.

The race was sponsored by the York Barbell Company, that company's president, Bob Hoffman, being an enthusiastic supporter of amateur sports: not just weight lifting at the Olympic level, but also road racing. Hoffman, ahead of his time, believed runners might benefit from strength training. In addition to a bronze medal hung from a red-white-and-blue ribbon, my third place award was an 80-pound set of barbells. Had I been traveling by plane, it probably would have been both difficult and expensive to transport my prize home. Fortunately, Browning drove me back to Philadelphia and helped load the weights into the baggage car of my return train.

Thus did I receive my introduction to strength training.

That's only partially true. As a track athlete in college, I did calisthenics—pushups, situps—as part of my warmup. Before being drafted into the U.S. Army, I did a lot of both to prepare myself for the rigors of basic training. I still take pride in the fact that I was able to do more situps than any other soldier in my company: 80 in a period of 2 minutes during a physical fitness test. But until I won the York barbells, I never had done any serious weight lifting before. That was for bodybuilders and football players, I thought, not track athletes.

My position on the importance of strength training has changed. If you absorb only a single message from this book, it is that strength training is essential for success as a masters runner. If you never have done any weight training before, it is not too late to start. If you already lift weights to improve or maintain fitness, keep doing it. Research by William J. Evans, Ph.D., at Tufts University in Boston suggested that people in their eighties and nineties, women as well as men, could significantly improve their bone density and overall strength if they started to lift weights. If they could lift with some intensity, that was even better.

"One of the important benefits of strength training for masters runners," claims Dr. Evans, currently at the University of Arkansas, "is that it greatly strengthens the knee, hip, and ankle joints and may decrease the risk of orthopedic injuries."

Certainly, many more options exist today for strength training than did when I brought that 80-pound set of barbells home from

York, Pennsylvania. You can purchase home exercise equipment at the local shopping mall or join a health club that offers dozens of exercise machines, each focusing

> If you absorb only a single message from this book, it is that strength training is essential for success as a masters runner.

on a different body part. Whereas gyms once were the domain of muscle-bound males, featherweight females now have no fears of pumping iron. While in Florida, my wife, Rose, participates in regular strength classes, both in a pool and in an exercise room. In its exercise guidelines, originally developed under the direction of Michael L. Pollock, Ph.D., the American College of Sports Medicine preaches that strength training at least twice a week is essential for longevity and good health.

In my book *Run Fast,* written more than a decade ago, I identified three groups that might best benefit from strength training: (1) ectomorphs, (2) women, and (3) masters. Ectomorphs are skinny people like me, those most likely to have had sand kicked in their faces by the bullies at the beach. Women tend to have less muscle mass than men, but can improve it through strength training. Those likely to suffer from osteoporosis as they age (the skinniest women) need to lift weight to improve and maintain bone density. Masters definitely need to pump some iron. In *Run Fast,* I quoted Dr. Pollock as saying, "Strength fades as we age. As strength fades, so does speed."

STRENGTH FADES FASTER THAN ENDURANCE

Dr. Pollock explained that this was easily measurable in exercise laboratories and that strength faded faster than endurance, one reason why older runners have more success against younger runners in ultramarathons than in 1500-meter races. I notice that as I age, I find it increasingly difficult in road races to match the pace of runners near me going uphill. I may catch them on the downhill and move away on the flat, but on uphills, I lose ground. Most certainly this is because of diminished strength in the quadriceps muscles, essential for raising the knees during each uphill stride. "As you get older, you need to focus more and more on the strength aspect of your conditioning," said Dr. Pollock. I do, and always have, but I would be the first to admit that it is not always easy and convenient to devote even an extra 30 to 60 minutes a week to strength training.

Following my return from York, I used my third-place barbells to work out on the back porch of my apartment on the south side of Chicago. I also did weight lifting in the gym at the University of Chicago where I ran track workouts. Coach Ted Haydon usually steered his runners away from the weight room, but I was as much interested in pleasure as performance. If you enjoy exercise, lifting weights can be fun. Without any specific coaching, I simply mimicked the three lifts used in the Olympics, trying to lift as much as I could shove overhead. But I soon became bored with the routine and within a few years donated the weights to Mount Carmel High School, where I coached part-time for several years. This happened during a period where I had begun to push my weekly training miles up past 100. Not only did I not have much time to devote to extra training, but I did not have enough extra energy. As an elite runner, you often need more sleep to recover from the hard training you do. Today's full-time, professional runners can afford the extra time necessary to do supplemental exercises, but elites form only a small percentage of the running population. The rest of us need to think creatively to be able to fit strength training into our already busy lives.

In the late 1970s, I appeared at a clinic sponsored by *Runner's World* in California, where one of the other speakers was Bill Reynolds, a weight lifter who had written *The Complete Weight Training Book.* Talks with Bill convinced me that I should resume lifting. This was during a period in my life when I was running nowhere near the 100 weekly miles of my elite youth, so I had both the time and energy. He suggested five basic barbell lifts, which I use to this day (see "Barbells" on page 161).

In the mid-1980s, we remodeled the basement of our home in Long Beach, Indiana. My article detailing the planning and construction of a "runner's basement" appeared in the April 1984 issue

BARBELLS

Strength training can be cheap and easy if you own a barbell. When I first started to supplement my running with weight lifting, I used the classic Olympic lifts. I also listened to Nautilus instructors whose machine-based approach was to lift to muscle exhaustion. But, as a runner, I wasn't interested in bulking up. The tight abs and six-packs now promoted in magazines such as *Men's Health* remained far from my main focus. Runners benefit most by workouts that combine light weights and high repetitions.

The five basic exercises taught me in 1978 by weight lifter Bill Reynolds that I described in *Run Fast* still make sense to me today.

1. **Clean and press.** An Olympic lift. Stand with feet spread, reach down, grasp the bar, and bring it overhead in one continuous motion. Repeat the full movement a dozen or so times.

2. **Bent-over row.** Knees slightly bent, grasp the bar palms down. Lift to your chest without rising from the bent position. Repeat.

3. **Upright row.** Palms down, grasp the bar and stand straight, lifting the bar thigh high. With elbows out, now lift the bar chest high. Repeat.

4. **Curl.** Standing upright, palms out, elbows close to your body, lift the bar toward your shoulders. Repeat.

5. **Military press.** Again upright, palms down, bring the bar to shoulder height, then raise it repeatedly overhead.

How often should you repeat each lift? That depends on how much time you want to devote to lifting. I usually repeat each lift a dozen times, stretch briefly, then shift to the next lift. I never pay much attention to how much weight I place on the bar. I lift enough to tax my muscles without maxing them out. I approach strength training the way I now approach running: Whatever works on any particular day, works.

of *The Runner* magazine immediately before the Boston Marathon that year. It seemed like every runner I met that race weekend had read the article and commented how mine had become their fantasy basement. Central to planning the basement was consulting with an architect, Doug Wickstrom, who analyzed my movements before and after each run. This dictated where we located the shower; a whirlpool; shelves for clothes and shoes; and even a cork wall to which I could attach posters, race numbers, and a calendar to record my mileage. There also was space, beside the laundry area, for strength-training equipment.

In addition to barbells, I acquired a Total Gym, actually a sliding bench with pulleys that permits you to use your own weight for resistance. Changing the angle of the bench allows you to increase the degree of difficulty. Although instructions that came with the Total Gym demonstrated several dozen different exercises, I focused only on a few, including several that strengthened the same arm and shoulder muscles used in cross-country skiing. Essential to any strength-training program is figuring out a routine that works for you, one that motivates you enough to continue. Fall short of that goal, and you'll have a more difficult time pushing yourself to do the necessary training.

During a 1995 lecture tour through the Southwest, while promoting one of my books, I spoke to the Oklahoma City Running Club and spent a night as guest of runners Bonnie and Cullen Thomas. They had an exercise room that included a HealthRider, a machine that you ride like a motorcycle, pulling with your arms and pushing with your legs. Bonnie used the HealthRider as part of her fitness routine and offered a demonstration. After returning home, I acquired the machine, eventually giving the Total Gym away.

But you don't require a large basement or need to spend a lot of money, either on home equipment or membership in a health club, to strength-train. Dumbbells are relatively cheap and occupy little space. You can even use them while watching TV. One day I noticed that the plastic jugs of liquid Tide we used for our laundry had handles that made them easy to grip. Filled with 100 fluid ounces of water apiece, they weighed 6.25 pounds each and made effective dumbbells. I use them now mainly in a swinging motion that mimics the running armswing, but they also can be used to do presses and curls and other exercises you might do in any health club.

THE NEW-TIME GYM

In 1999, our second son, David, moved his family from Portland, Oregon, to Jacksonville, Florida. This conveniently came at a time when Rose and I were seeking a second home in a warm clime. The fact that two of our grandchildren now lived in Florida offered an excuse to purchase a condo in Ponte Vedra Beach only a few minutes' walk from the ocean and a beach whose hard-packed sand at low tide offered the almost perfect surface for running. I noticed almost immediately the benefit to my aged knees. Another benefit of our location was access to The Lodge & Club, which included in its membership perks a heated, outdoor pool for lap swimming and a room packed with exercise equipment. We acquired a membership, the availability of all that equipment defining a new strength-training routine for me.

My visits in previous decades to gyms where weight lifters worked out had not always motivated me to continue. Old-time gyms often smelled bad, looked bad, and seemed inhospitable to those whose priorities didn't include training for the Mr. Universe contest.

New-time gyms, however, provide a more hospitable environment for individuals such as myself whose goals are more fitness related. They are brightly lit with sparkling exercise machines. This certainly describes The Lodge's fitness center, which typically has more women than men using the facilities, at least during the morning hours when my wife and I normally appear.

But even a new-time gym can prove frightening if you are not used to the environment. All those machines: How do you use them? Recently, when The Lodge's fitness center closed for remodeling, and I was forced to shift my workouts to another center owned by the same corporation a mile and a half down the beach, I did not feel comfortable with the different layout of machines and the different people I saw using them. I felt relieved after the re-modeling ended and I could return to my old health haunts. Admittedly, we are all creatures of habit.

> Essential to any strength-training program is figuring out a routine that works for you.

When I first began using the fitness center, I looked for assistance to Cathy Vasto, a friend who had competed in the 5000 meters at the Olympic trials on three separate occasions. (Vasto's personal record for that distance is 15:38.) When we first met, Cathy was working part-time as a personal trainer to supplement her income as a runner. She helped me devise a basic workout routine that we eventually modified and offered, complete with demonstration photos featuring Cathy, on my Web site. "Runners need to improve their speed," Cathy Vasto advised, "and one of the best ways to do that is with strength training."

Here are some of Vasto's recommendations.

High/low. If you're training for a race, you don't want to bulk up. Extra weight will slow you down. To avoid putting on pounds, keep the weight you lift low and the repetitions high. Vasto recommends lifting 50 to 60 percent of the maximum weight you can lift in a set of 12 repetitions. If you have time, repeat the set. For maximum benefits, do your strength training two or three times a week, after you run, not before.

Look good lifting. Keep your form—not for vanity, but to prevent injury. Think 90 degrees. Most seated lifts work best if your body parts are at right angles: legs straight, feet flat against the floor, trunk erect, chin up, eyes forward. Practice the pelvic tilt where you press your torso back against the chair or floor to keep your back from slumping. "Good form works in lifting as much as it does in running," says Vasto.

Breathe right. The worst mistake you can make while lifting is to hold your breath. That simply tightens the muscles that you want to keep loose. Inhale while you prepare to lift the weight, then exhale while lifting it, inhaling again while lowering it. "The best way to breathe is naturally," says Vasto, "so that you're not even aware you're doing it."

Rest by stretching. When moving from exercise to exercise, don't rush, and don't waste time chitchatting with friends. Stay focused on your workout by stretching in between. "It's very important while strength training to have a stretching routine," warns Vasto. "You don't want to lose your flexibility, which can happen if you forget to stretch. Eccentric contractions (which occur when lowering the weights) actually can tighten the muscles." Stretching while doing your strength training provides a double dose of conditioning in a minimum of time.

THE PERSONAL TRAINER

The half-dozen basic strength-training exercises suggested by Cathy Vasto got me started at The Lodge (see "Lifts for the Gym" on page 166). At a later date, when I wanted to expand my routine, I sought the advice of another personal trainer who worked at The Lodge's fitness center: Greg McDaniels. Seeking help is always a good idea. After joining a new fitness center, if not familiar with the equipment, you probably need to ask someone to escort you through the gym and point out each machine and describe its uses. Many health clubs provide this service to their members. But sometimes you can benefit from a refresher course and thus need to hire a personal trainer to conduct a walk-through.

Why is this important? The trainer can actually show you how to use the equipment and correct your form if you are not lifting correctly. "Once you commit the time to the gym," suggests McDaniels, "you will be able to train much more efficiently if you get somebody to teach you good posture and correct biomechanics. With poor technique, you dramatically increase your chance of injury."

Most exercise machines are well designed and somewhat foolproof, but you will get the best results from your strength training if you perform the lifts correctly. Consider also the possibility of hiring a personal trainer to work with you on a regular basis one or more times a week. The most important reason to do so would be for

(continued on page 168)

LIFTS FOR THE GYM

When she worked as a personal trainer at The Lodge & Club in Ponte Vedra Beach, Florida, Olympic trials 5000-meter runner Cathy Vasto showed me how to do a half-dozen strength-training exercises, which I later featured on my Web site. "Strength is important for masters runners," claims Vasto, "not only to improve your speed for running races, but it will make you feel good and look good and improve the quality of your life, throughout your lifetime."

Here are the half-dozen strength-training exercises recommended by Cathy Vasto.

Bench press. This is a basic lift, used by all bodybuilders, but you can use it to build strength and speed. Lie on your back on a bench. For weight, use a barbell or dumbbells. Keep your back flat, your knees bent. Your palms should be facing forward, your hands should be equally distant to and over your shoulders. Lift the bar or dumbbells straight up (think 90 degrees), and lower slowly. For an alternate workout without weights, do simple pushups. The bench press strengthens the pectorals, deltoids, triceps, and biceps.

Rowing. Gripping dumbbells, sit on the edge of a bench or firm chair, keeping your back straight. Hold the dumbbells with your arms extended, palms facing inward against your knees. Raise the dumbbells to just opposite your chest, then return to the starting position. You can also do this exercise while standing, keeping your knees bent at a 45-degree angle and your torso bent forward. Another option is to use a single weight gripped in both hands, and bring it up to your chest. Rowing strengthens the rhomboids.

Overhead pull. "This is an easy exercise," says Vasto. "You can do it with a 16-ounce can of soup, a 5-pound bag of flour, or a water bottle if you don't have a dumbbell. The angle multiplies the effect of even light weights." Take the object and hold it overhead, elbows forward, back straight, knees slightly bent to take the pressure off your back. (You can also do this exercise while seated.) Lower the weight behind your head toward the back of your neck, then return to the starting position. The overhead pull strengthens the triceps.

Curl. Sit in a chair, feet flat on the floor, stomach in, shoulders back, head up. Your elbows should be against your waist above your hips, your palms up holding the weights. Raise the weights to your shoulders, lowering slowly. "Two cans of soup work as well as barbells or dumbbells," claims Vasto. This exercise can also be done standing up. Curls strengthen the biceps.

Crunch. Unlike the other five exercises, this is not a lift, but Vasto recommends crunches, because they isolate the abdominal muscles. "The abs are your core of balance," she says. "They support your upper body, important at the end of a race." (A crunch is a situp where you stop after raising your shoulders off the floor.) In the starting position, your back should be flat against the floor, your head up, eyes on the ceiling, hands gripping the back of your neck, your knees relaxed and bent, feet on the floor. Raise only to the point where you feel your stomach muscles tightening, hold, then release, returning your back to the floor. Crunches strengthen the abdominal muscles, referred to as the abs.

Lunge. The five previous exercises strengthen the upper body, often neglected by runners. The lunge will help strengthen several of the muscles of the lower body. Start this exercise with your feet shoulder-width apart. If you use a barbell, it should rest across your shoulders and behind your neck. If using dumbbells, hold them beside your thighs. If not used to this exercise, you should begin first without weights. Take a long step forward with one leg and descend to a low position, then rise. Bring the lead leg back, and repeat with the other leg forward. Form is very important in doing this exercise to avoid injury. "Again, think 90 degrees," warns Vasto. The lunge strengthens many of the muscles of the legs, including the quadriceps, hamstrings, gluteals, and erector spinae.

motivation, in short supply with many individuals. If you're looking to save time, if not money, you can hire a personal trainer to work with you in your home.

Each winter when we return to Florida, I get a refresher course from McDaniels or one of the other trainers at The Lodge's fitness center. Since my summer training in Indiana often differs from my winter training in Florida, it permits me to reestablish a rhythm in my workouts. Also, my training goals may differ from year to year, suggesting a modified approach. Recently, when The Lodge remodeled its fitness center, bringing in entirely new machines, I found the help of a trainer necessary to point out the pluses and minuses of each one, at least for meeting my own particular goals.

I don't use every exercise machine. With several dozen machines available, doing so would stretch my workout past the 15 or 30 minutes I want to spend in the weight room. I wander from machine to machine in no particular order, not always using the same machine from workout to workout. That way, I don't have to stand waiting while some other individual finishes using the machine I want to use.

Nevertheless, I do follow a certain pattern, beginning most often with dumbbells. I select a light pair of dumbbells and move through a set of four or five lifts similar to those suggested by Cathy Vasto. Sitting on the edge of the bench, I do presses and curls, then lie down and do presses from a horizontal position, finally doing side lifts where I hold the dumbbells overhead, then lower them so my arms are straight out from my body, parallel to the ground, at a 90-degree angle from my torso. If there's an approved name to this exercise, I don't know it. It just feels good to me, and that may be the most important reason to do it.

I'll do about a dozen repeats of each lift, then stand beside the bench and swing the dumbbells with my arms in a motion similar to running. I replace those dumbbells in the rack and pick up the next heaviest set, repeating the same routine. Then I look around to see what machines are open. Ideally, I prefer following an upper-body exercise with a lower-body exercise, stretching between. No specific stretch; just whatever comes to mind. McDaniels emphasizes that it is important to warm up before stretching. "You need to get your core body temperature up," he says. "Cold muscles too easily become injured."

Runners need to improve their speed, and one of the best ways to do that is with strength training.

McDaniels suggests a 5-minute walk as prelude. If I haven't already run on the beach, I'll sometimes jump onto a treadmill to walk and jog for 10 minutes before starting to lift.

Continuing my routine, I often move from the dumbbells to a nearby body press machine that allows more serious weight lifters to load the bar with as many pounds as they want. I'm usually content to lift the bar alone, and it irritates me if someone using the machine previously has left heavy weights attached to the bar, a definite breach of weight room etiquette (see "Gym Etiquette" on page 170). Rather than remove the weights from the bar and risk a possible injury, I simply skip that machine and choose another.

Or I may do some floor exercises. Currently, I have two in my repertoire. The first involves a plastic ball, usually found tucked in a corner if someone from an exercise class hasn't borrowed it. Lying flat on the ground, I position my lower legs on top of the ball, my calves pressed against it, so my body forms two 90-degree angles at the knees and waist. My shoulders remaining pressed to the ground, I lift my torso, hold, and release. Greg has carefully coached me to lock my back and shoulders on the ground before each raise. Doing this doesn't come naturally, so I correct myself each time. After 15 or 20 raises (good for the abs), I kick the ball aside, lock my toes under a handy machine, and do some crunches, which are basically situps where you stop in the middle rather than continuing to touch your knees.

At the same end of the gym where the barbells are located is a pullup machine, one that allows you to use weights to balance your body weight and make it easier to do the pullups. There are three lifts that I do on the machine, two similar to the standard pullup but with the hands angled at different directions, and a third where the bar and your arms are below as you lift your body. Not being into

(continued on page 172)

GYM ETIQUETTE

Are you a stranger to strength training, afraid to push the glass door open to gain entry to that room with the mirrors and glitzy equipment? Fear not: Weight-lifting rooms once were the exclusive domain of sweaty males trying to max out their muscles. A gentler and friendlier environment exists today, with more and more women as well as older men using fitness centers to both get in and stay in shape. Here's how to behave when you walk into the gym.

Stay cool. Don't be self-conscious. You have as much right to be there as any over-muscled hulk or tightly toned female. They won't even notice you; they're too intent on their own mirrored reflections.

Forget fashion. You don't need to wear the latest spandex fashions to fit in. Billy Joel's proverbial "cheap pair of sneakers" will do. "Many people who go to a gym are intimidated by the cutting-edge clothing they see," says Ed Brickell of Dallas, "but uniforms are not necessary."

Don't try to compete. This means either with others in the gym or even yourself. It doesn't matter how much weight you put on the bar. Again, nobody cares. Your only purpose in a health club is to get strong, not to show off.

Get help. It's all right not to know everything about strength training the first day you arrive at the health club. "Many gyms offer introductory tours with a trainer," says Nancy Armour of Chicago. "You not only get to see what the different machines do, but how to use them."

Sweating is acceptable. What is not acceptable is sweating on the equipment and not wiping it off when you move to the next machine. That's why they hand you a towel before you enter. Amanda Musacchio of Villa Park, Illinois, adds: "Spitting is uncouth too, particularly on the floor."

Towels have double purposes. You can drape a towel over a bench briefly to reserve space while you fetch some extra weights. That's okay, but notice I said briefly. Don't hog equipment to the exclusion of others.

Cut the chatter. No rule exists that you can't engage in conversations with fellow exercisers, but limit socializing. "Some people take chatting to the extreme, where it becomes distracting and annoying," says Dan Schwartz of Boulder, Colorado. Lounging around on machines that others might want to use also is unacceptable.

Cut the noise, too. Letting the weights bang to the floor after lifting may make you feel manly, but the noise can startle and irritate other exercisers. Ken Fleck of Lombard, Illinois, adds: "Excessive grunting also can be intrusive."

Return weights after use. If you add more weights to a bar or machine, return those weights to the rack when done. The next exerciser may not want to pump as much iron as you, or may not be able to remove your heavy weights.

Be aware of others nearby. Don't move into their exercise space, actual or visual. If you inadvertently cause someone to drop a weight, it may land on your toe. This advice includes the locker room. "Other people need to share the benches, floor space, and clothes racks, too," says Deidre Wesley of Newburgh, Indiana.

Don't stink. Certain smells come with the territory, but don't add to them. "Avoid wearing excessive cologne or perfume," pleads Autumn Evans of Melbourne Beach, Florida. "Strong scents can be difficult to take while exercising vigorously."

Don't hog the equipment. This is particularly true with treadmills and other machines for which there may be people waiting. If there is a time limit, honor it. Run that final 20-miler outdoors.

It's not that difficult to survive in the weight room. Be aware that different fitness centers may have slightly different rules, both posted and understood. It may take you a few visits, and perhaps some guidance from a staff member or personal trainer, before you feel comfortable in the weight room, but strength training is a must for all masters runners.

brute strength, I usually set the weight at a medium level and use the exercise as much as a flexibility drill as for strengthening. This is a purpose similar to when I am home in Indiana and run to a nearby golf course. I always pause briefly to stretch beneath a tree, one of my favorite stretches being to grab an upper branch and hang from it. Particularly in the area of stretching, I am more inclined to invent my own stretches rather than follow routines described in books.

IS STRETCHING NECESSARY?

Trends in exercise change. When running first became a populist activity, we all were urged to stretch our muscles as both a preventive for injuries and for recovery if injured. This made sense to me. As a steeplechaser who needed the flexibility to hurdle 3-foot barriers, I already did what passed for stretching exercises, even though I never thought of them by that name. "Calisthenics" was a word that covered a lot of ground for those of us who preceded the running boom of the 1970s.

Unfortunately, there seemed to be little research that proved stretching could prevent injury. One study at the Honolulu Marathon actually suggested that those most injured stretched more than their noninjured brethren. (This may have been because they started to stretch only after becoming injured.) More off-putting when stretching first became popular, we were asked to stretch for such long periods of time (60 seconds) and to use so many different stretches (dozens of routines) that there hardly seemed time to run. My most vivid memory of excessive stretching was when I used to train on the 400-meter indoor track at the East Bank Club in downtown Chicago. I spotted one elegantly attired female stretching on the mats beside the track before I started to run, and she still was stretching after I headed to the showers. At least she looked good, which may have been her purpose for being there.

The current trend, suggests McDaniels, is "active isolated stretching," an approach promoted by Aaron Mattes of Stretching USA. According to Mattes: "Using a 2-second stretch has proven to be the key in avoiding reflexive contraction of the antagonistic

STRETCHING FOR SUCCESS

Debbie Pitchford is a physical therapist for Novacare and works at Medical Group Outpatient Rehabilitation in Michigan City, Indiana. As a physical therapist, Pitchford understands how to stretch correctly, something she claims not all runners know how to do. She offers the following advice for runners who want to increase their speed and prevent injuries by developing flexibility.

Warm up and cool down. Stretching is important during your warmup, before you run, because it increases bloodflow to the muscles. But stretching during your cooldown may be even more important. "After running,' stretching helps to remove lactic acid from the muscles, which in turn reduces muscle soreness," says Pitchford. "That promotes better flexibility." Stretching afterward also will help you relax.

Don't overstretch. While stretching can promote flexibility, stretching too far actually can damage the muscles—particularly if you're recovering from an injury. "A healthy muscle can elongate up to 1.6 times its length," suggests Pitchford, "but generally doesn't respond well to that much stretching." By overstretching, you create an automatic reflex that actually will cause the muscle to recoil to protect itself from tearing and injury. Also, don't bounce while stretching. Holding your stretch in a static position works best.

Combine stretching and strengthening. A good time to do your stretching exercises is while resting between lifts during your strength training. Strength training will not decrease your flexibility, says Pitchford, as long as you do it properly and perform your lifts through their full range of motion.

Pitchford believes it a myth that aging is the only factor that causes us to lose flexibility. "It's lack of exercise," she says. "Studies show that a sedentary lifestyle is a bigger factor in decreasing flexibility than aging." If you stay active aerobically and use stretching to maintain your flexibility, you will look and feel younger because of the way you move.

muscles." Is the Mattes quick-stretch approach better than previous methods that suggested holding stretches for 60 seconds or more? I'm not sure, but it sure makes sense for busy people, masters included.

Continuing my strength-training routine, several other machines allow me the opportunity to push or pull various weights. I pick whichever machines are vacant, at the same time eyeing the clock to

NANCY CLARK ON NUTRITION FOR MASTERS

Should masters runners eat differently from younger runners? Not according to Nancy Clark, R.D., senior sports nutritionist at Healthworks Fitness Center and author of *Nancy Clark's Sports Nutrition Guidebook*. "There are no major nutritional changes for masters athletes," states Clark.

However, older runners may need to make some minor nutritional changes, starting with a determination of whether or not you already are eating healthy. Regardless of what promoters of low-carb and various other fad diets say, endurance athletes should make 55 percent carbohydrates, 30 percent fats, and 15 percent proteins their nutritional goal. Distrust any food that comes wrapped in plastic, and balance your diet with plenty of fresh fruits, vegetables, and whole grains. Red meat is not necessarily bad, since it contains iron, zinc, and B vitamins. Also, for those who like me had a Catholic grade-school education, when the nuns told us to eat fish on Fridays, they had the right idea. Particularly, salmon, swordfish, and tuna are rich in oils necessary for heart health. Pasta the night before a marathon? It's the perfect meal.

In her column "The Athlete's Kitchen," Clark analyzed the different food groups and what masters should focus on when eating.

Carbohydrates. "Multigrain bagels, rye crackers, brown rice, and oatmeal are just a few examples of wholesome grain foods that both fuel muscles and protect against cancer, diabetes, and heart disease," writes Clark. She also promotes carbohydrate-rich bananas, orange juice, and yogurt smoothies. All promote quick recovery after races and workouts.

Protein. As we age, our protein needs increase slightly, claims Clark,

make sure I don't spend more than the 15 or so minutes I have allocated that day for strength training. Two lower-leg machines I always use involve lifting weights seated or prone. These strengthen the muscles around the knees, including the hamstrings, and are important for preventing knee injuries. Following Greg's advice, I do not overload the machines with heavy weights. Similar to Cathy Vasto, he prefers that I use relatively light weights, but maintain good form

but no reason exists for different recommendations. Eat protein with at least two meals per day. Clark pushes peanut butter on toast, turkey sandwiches on multigrain bread, and spaghetti with meat sauce. Vegetarians need to focus on beans, nuts, and soy plus other protein-rich plant food. Introduce yourself to hummus and tofu.

Fat. Healthful plant and fish oils, says Clark, have a health-protective anti-inflammatory effect. She writes: "Given that diseases of aging, such as heart disease and diabetes, are thought to be triggered by inflammation, consuming plant and fish oils that reduce inflammation is a wise choice." Eat peanut butter five or more times per week, and you reduce your risk of heart disease by 21 percent. That legitimizes the peanut-butter-and-jelly sandwiches I love. Married to an Italian wife, I fall easily into the role of mixing marvelous salads topped with olive oil. I've always considered super-low-fat diets (15 percent or less) hazardous to health.

Nancy Clark also recommends that masters runners select foods that contain calcium (milk, yogurt, cheese) to maintain bone strength. Fiber such as that found in whole grain cereals and oatmeal reduces cholesterol and allows for regular bowel movements. Do you need extra vitamins and other supplements? Not according to Nancy. A daily multivitamin offers a good hedge against deficiency, but unless your physician has other ideas, you should be able to obtain all the vitamins and minerals you need by eating properly. Also, the more you exercise, the more you eat, allowing you to consume more vitamins from fresh foods.

"Eat wisely, drink plenty of fluids, exercise regularly, lift weights, refuel rapidly, and enjoy feeling young," recommends Clark. Masters runners don't need fad diets; they need a sensible approach to food.

rather than straining. I notice that when others use the same machines, they often lift with painful looks on their faces, accompanying their exercises with ugly grunts. I want to keep the lifting easy enough so I can smile, if necessary. This is similar to my philosophy for easy runs. One way to judge if you're running too fast is whether or not you can comfortably carry on a conversation with a training partner.

Nevertheless, I try to avoid conversations while lifting weights. I see other individuals working with their personal trainer who often carry on a steady conversation on subjects totally unrelated to the exercises they are doing. That's fine if your object is relaxation and an opportunity to communicate with another individual. I do this while seated in a barber chair when someone else is doing all the work, but never while pumping iron. I want to focus on what I'm doing, just as I never carry on a conversation with other runners while trying to run fast or while competing in a race.

9 ERRORS

If You Want to Succeed as a Masters Runner, Make Sure You Never Get Injured

During the summer of 1983, I visited Washington, D.C., on business and decided to contact friends who lived in the city: Bill and Jackie O'Neil. My wife, Rose, accompanied me on the trip. We decided to go canoeing Saturday on Chesapeake Bay. The day was warm. The sun shone in a cloudless sky. A light breeze cooled us. We paused from paddling to sip some wine and eat a picnic lunch. We hadn't seen the O'Neils in more than a decade, so the day turned into a memorable outing. Somehow it didn't occur to me—or maybe I didn't care—that sitting cramped in a canoe might not be the best preparation for a race scheduled the next day.

Sunday, I planned to run the 1500 meters in a masters track meet in Virginia. Bill and Jackie came along to see me run. Somewhat stiff from the previous day's canoeing, I warmed up carefully: jogging, stretching, bounding, then cruised a 200 on the back straightaway. I knew that the shorter the race distance, the more attention I needed to give my warmup. Waiting for the start, however, I felt something pop in my left leg below the knee. Not a pull, more a strain. I continued my warmup, but although I could run, it was painful to run fast. I aborted my race plans and departed the track.

Three weeks later, despite regular doses of ice and aspirin, I still could not run comfortably. An orthopedist diagnosed my injury as a calf pull and recommended inserts. The injury hardly proved career-threatening, but was serious enough to put a damper on my preparations for the World Masters Championships in Puerto Rico a few months later. I cancelled plans to compete, partly because of the injury, partly because work on a book had begun to absorb a lot of my time and attention. We scheduled a research trip to Italy instead of a running trip to Puerto Rico. In all honesty, the injury offered me an excuse to skip the track meet in a year when masters competition had slipped two or three notches on my priority list.

Looking back on my running career, however, if I could undo one decision, it would be that one. For the remainder of the summer, I rehabilitated by swimming and jogging in deep water and pedaling an exercise bike in my basement. I walked and jogged on soft grass when possible. I listened to my body. If the leg hurt, I slowed down or stopped. By the end of August, I was "cured." At the Park Forest Scenic Ten in Illinois on Labor Day, I placed first in the 50–54 age group. A month later, I won a 4-mile cross-country race in South Bend, Indiana, overall against younger runners.

But I missed what was the Fifth World Masters Championships in Puerto Rico in 1983, no big deal at the time, except more than 2 decades later it is the only World Masters Championships I have missed! Before the 10th championships in Miyazaki, Japan, in 1993, the organizers decided to honor those individuals who had run all ten. My name appeared on an initial list of those being honored, but I had to beg out of the ceremony. Despite being entered at Puerto Rico, I had not run. At the most recent championships, held again in Puerto Rico in 2003, the number of those who had competed in all 15 meets had shrunk to eight individuals. I will forever be one short of being able to join that elite group onstage.

Injuries seem almost inevitable if you want to succeed as a masters runner. They are a sword of Damocles hovering over our heads each time we attempt to motivate

> Show me a masters runner who never has been injured, and I'll show you a runner who is suffering from serious denial.

ourselves for success. In order to achieve peak performance, you need to train hard. You need to increase your weekly mileage, particularly if training for a marathon. You need to add speedwork to your training routine if training for shorter distances such as the 5-K or 10-K. You need to run when the weather is too cold or too hot or too windy or too rainy and when there is snow or ice on the

STREAKERS

Only eight athletes competed in the first 15 World Masters Championships between 1975 and 2003. A ninth, Hari Chandra, a 400-meter runner from Singapore, attended all championships as an officer of the World Masters Association; however, he did not always compete. These are the streakers.

Ruth Anderson, USA: long-distance runner

Reg Austin, Australia: sprinter

John Dunsford, Great Britain: racewalker; shot-putter

Willie Dunne, Ireland: long-distance runner

Bob Fine, USA: racewalker

Bob Mimm, USA: racewalker

Jim O'Neil, USA: long-distance runner

Jack Stevens, Australia: middle-distance runner

Not only has Jim O'Neil of Rancho Mirage, California, competed in every World Masters Championships, he also has competed in every USA Masters Championships, beginning with 1971, the only athlete to have done so. "Just to be counted among this elite group is an honor," says O'Neil, who has won a dozen world titles, including road races. "I didn't start out with a plan to outlast all the other runners. It just happened that way, but I now admit not wanting to break the string is a factor in keeping me going."

ground and at odd times of the day, when it is too dark to see, and over uneven surfaces, because even the smoothest road has potholes that can swallow an unwary runner. Show me a masters runner who never has been injured, and I'll show you a runner who is suffering from serious denial.

Most running injuries are not life-threatening; they simply keep us from doing what we love to do, which is to run.

A HANDFUL OF INJURIES

A frequent question asked me by younger runners who hope some day to become older runners is: "How often have you been injured?" Not too often, I admit. And that in a running career that began in 1947 and has spanned 7 decades. Other than the 1983 injury that forced me to abort my plans to compete in the Worlds that year, only two other injuries proved serious enough to cause me to miss more than a week or two of training.

Funny that no matter how much memory fades as we age, certain moments stand out with such crystal clarity that it is almost like popping a DVD into your digital player: You recall every sight, sound, and smell. That second and most serious injury occurred in 1970 at the end of a workout on a cinder track at the junior high school near my home in Long Beach. I wasn't keeping a training diary at that time, but I suspect I had just run something like 12 × 440 yards, jogging 440 between, a classic interval workout. Running with me that day were several runners from Chesterton High School, including a freshman named Steve Wynder, who would win the state title in cross-country his senior year.

Finishing the final quarter, we paused to chat. What was the cause of what happened next? I was fatigued from a hard workout. The weather was cool. The junior-high track was barely better than a gravel pit, its looseness certainly stressing our muscles more than usual. I don't know how many miles I had run or how hard I had trained in the days and weeks before that single workout. Was overtraining a factor? Probably. Age? I was only 39 years old, not yet a master. Perhaps we talked too long, and my muscles stiffened. Someone said, "Let's jog a few laps to cool down."

POP!

I didn't even get my foot off the ground to take the first step. My brain sent a message to the body to start running, and the body protested by snapping something in one knee. "You're not running another step," the body told the brain. I needed to be driven home. I immediately made an appointment to see an orthopedic surgeon. I feared that I had torn cartilage, which would necessitate arthroscopic surgery, but such was not the case. A ligament or tendon (I forget which) was severely strained, not torn. Although I needed to use crutches for nearly a month and could not run for still another month, the injury eventually healed itself, and I was able to run again.

The third and final major injury was a stress fracture that occurred in a way that few reading this book will experience. Over a period of years, my close friend Steve Kearney and I had discussed the possibility of running the length of the state of Indiana: 350 miles from Owensboro, Kentucky (my father's birthplace), to Michiana Shores, Michigan (a mile up the road from my home in Long Beach). We recruited a total of 10 runners to participate in what we called the Trans Indiana Run, not a race but more a test of wills. (I described the event in an article titled "The Indy 350" in the November 1985 issue of *The Runner*, later reprinted in John Parker's 1991 book about ultramarathoning, *And Then the Vulture Eats You*.)

Midway through the 10-day run, one ankle started to ache, forcing me into an ice-and-aspirin routine in order to be able to continue. Curiously, I found that the faster I ran, the better the ankle felt. The shortest distance we ran was on the ninth day, "only" 20 miles. Fellow lunatic Rich Breiner and I raced it at faster than a 7:00 pace. But halfway through the 25-mile 10th and final day, I felt a sudden twinge in a lower leg coming down an incline on a bridge over the Indiana toll road. I finished, but the next day podiatrist Mann Spittler, D.P.M., diagnosed the injury as a

> The way to prevent injuries from happening is to not make training errors.

DR. JOHN PAGLIANO ON RUNNING INJURIES

In a continuing clinical study of more than 4,000 runners he has seen in his Long Beach, California, offices, John W. Pagliano, D.P.M., suggests five reasons for running injuries, in this order.

1. **Training methods.** "The most common cause of running injuries is the failure to train properly," says Dr. Pagliano. "We commonly call this 'too much too soon.'" Dr. Pagliano quotes Stan James, M.D., writing in the *American Journal of Sports Medicine* that more than 50 percent of running injuries are due to training errors. Dr. Pagliano adds: "Excessive intensity and duration does not allow for proper physiological adaptation. The muscle and tendon structures fatigue easily, and overuse injuries occur." Failure to allow for a day of rest between hard training sessions is the most common training error.

2. **Training surfaces.** "The harder the surface, the more shock enters the lower extremity," says Dr. Pagliano. Pavement, obviously, is harder than trails or most tracks, but concrete also is harder than asphalt. "Transitioning from one type of surface to another can produce problems," says Dr. Pagliano. "If this is done gradually, there is little chance of injury."

stress fracture. I rehabilitated for 3 weeks with strength training, indoor cycling, and walking and resumed running in time to participate on a 4 × 800 relay team that set an M50 record of 9:06:41 at the National Masters Championships in Indianapolis. My time was relatively slow, but with Russ Bonham, Bill Heck, and Dick Wilson, I had three other fast runners to carry me.

Each injury taught me a valuable lesson, allowing me to run more safely in its aftermath. The lesson I learned from Trans Indiana was not to cram 350 miles of running into a period of 10 days. The calf pull that eliminated me from the 1983 World Championships certainly was the result of canoeing the day before a track meet. I normally would not have expected an interval workout on the track in

3. **Muscle dysfunction and inflexibility.** Running utilizes the same motions over and over and over. Dr. Pagliano advises: "Runners tend to be extremely inflexible, due to the repetitive nature of the sport. Regular stretching needs to be initiated at the introduction of the running program."

4. **Shoe design.** Today's running shoes are much more sophisticated than those available in decades past, but you need someone to tell you which shoe models work best for both your stride and size. Specialty running stores have become adept at performing gait analysis by watching their customers run on in-store treadmills or out the front door, but few shoe clerks have podiatry degrees. Worn or old shoes can cause problems, suggesting that runners need to check wear frequently and replace shoes that have too much mileage on them.

5. **Biomechanics of running.** "Runners with various lower-extremity malalignments will develop biomechanical or overuse injuries," warns Dr. Pagliano. Inserts can help correct minor problems; otherwise, orthotics crafted by a podiatrist may be a necessary option.

1970 to have caused such a severe knee injury, but perhaps I had been overtraining. Stan James, M.D., an orthopedic surgeon from Eugene, Oregon, suggests: "Most injuries are the result of training errors." I agree, and if I can teach you how to avoid those training errors based on my experience, it will help you become a better masters runner.

TRAINING ERRORS

Other than those three major injuries cited above, most of my injuries have been minor, ones that may have caused temporary pain, but little disruption in my training. Sometimes, however, they have limited my ability to compete as well as anticipated. Injuries can sometimes affect you psychologically as well as physically. For that reason, injuries should be avoided, and they can be avoided if you approach both your racing and training judiciously. Achieving this does take experience. It takes years to master the techniques of injury avoidance. That's an appropriate remark, because I suspect mas-

THE KNEES HAVE IT

It's a common question thrust at runners: "Don't your knees hurt?" Well, yeah, if I had a hard workout yesterday, but after an easy day or two, I'm ready to fly.

But the questioner doesn't want that answer. He wants to hear how badly we suffer each time we run. That gives him an excuse not to exercise in any form. "People often tell me my knees are going to be bad because of my running," sighs Lori Hauswirth of Merrill, Wisconsin. "I hear it most often from my mother."

Do runners suffer from knee problems as much as nonrunners think? In my survey of masters runners, 30 percent admitted to having suffered a knee injury. But how severe was that knee injury? Curious, I used the Inter*Active* Training Forum I manage online to question more than 300 runners about their knee problems. Among those responding, more than half suggested they suffered knee pain "infrequently." Another quarter of respondents reported knee pain "occasionally," while an equal number reported no knee pain. Only one runner, Jeff Schneller of Brookline, Massachusetts, who also identified himself as a downhill skier, confessed to continuous knee pain when he ran.

"My knees only seem to hurt after the mileage increases on a pair of shoes," admits Doug Richter of Vernon Hills, Illinois. "I always use this as a signal to replace the shoes."

In an article in the *Montreal Gazette* titled "The Joints Can Take It," Jill Barker suggests that exercises such as running actually strengthen the joints. "The stress of impact causes the joint to adapt positively, thereby improving its overall health," writes Barker. "There is, however, a threshold that if surpassed exceeds the normal wear and tear a joint can endure."

ters runners probably suffer fewer and lesser injuries than our younger counterparts. That's because we possess wisdom. Years of training have taught us how to train and how not to train. In this respect, the most useful tool for a masters runner trying to avoid injury is a diary of past training.

Determining a level of safe exercise, however, puzzles researchers. One study quoted by Barker suggests 55 weekly miles as the point where joint breakdown begins, but only a small percentage of runners train that much, even when getting ready for a marathon. Reportedly, if you limit your training to 15 to 25 miles a week, you're safe. A 1995 study at the Stanford University School of Medicine compared older runners with sedentary people and found that the runners reported less knee pain.

Increase mileage gradually, avoid gut-busting workouts, and you not only will spare your knees, but also the rest of your body. Intelligent training, not anti-inflammatories, is the best antidote for knee problems. "My knees bothered me when I first started running high mileage a dozen years ago," says Michele Keane of Westlake, Ohio, "but once I started strength training, they have not been a problem."

Keane pushed from 25 to 75 weekly miles in a matter of months after college to score a sub-3-hour marathon, but a side effect was sore knees. Years later after the birth of a child, she went from 0 to 50 miles for another marathon, using one of my training programs, with no knee pain. "The difference was a much gentler mileage increase," she reports.

Chip Loney was told never to run again after ACL (anterior cruciate ligament) reconstructive surgery to repair a basketball injury. He followed that advice for a decade, then started running again 3 years ago. "This year I will run Boston as my second marathon," says Loney. "My knee actually feels better now that I am running on a consistent basis than it did when I was not very active."

What, thus, should be your response the next time a nonrunner asks if your knees hurt? Smart-aleck replies won't do. Miss Manners would suggest a pleasant smile followed by, "My knees feel fine. How about you?"

Looking back through my training diaries, it seems that every third or fourth year I would suffer either plantar fascia or Achilles tendon problems, my two most common injuries. (As I write this chapter, I am just recovering from the latter injury.) These injuries, admittedly minor, most often have been related to my running the 3000-meter steeplechase, a high-stress event that involves hurdling four barriers and one water jump a lap. Plantar fasciitis can be particularly painful. It feels like someone has taken a hammer and whacked the bottom of your heel. Actually, the injury is a form of tendinitis of the tendon that stretches along the arch of the foot from ball to heel. The pain comes at the point where the tendon connects to the heel. When hurdling barriers or leaping the water jump in the steeplechase, you typically push off from the ball of your foot. If not properly warmed up, or if your foot muscles are stiff from over-training or fatigue, this pushing motion can cause you to stretch the fascia, or tendon. Running hills, which also forces you up on the balls of your feet, also can cause this injury. Steven Subotnick, D.P.M., a podiatrist from Hayward, California, once told me: "I see a lot of plantar fascia injuries, because there are so many hills near here." Runners who train on treadmills also risk plantar fasciitis if they raise the treadmill to too steep an angle.

Years past, on the occasions when I suffered a plantar fasciitis injury, my podiatrist would often tape the foot, effectively immobilizing the tendon so that it would not continue to stretch, allowing it time to heal. Today with mild cases of plantar fasciitis, podiatrists would be more likely to craft a heel pad to fit in a shoe. When runners who participate in the Inter*Active* Training forums I manage online ask questions about plantar fascia injuries, my first word of advice is to keep a pair of running shoes beside the bed and never get out of bed without putting on your shoes. The body is stiffest early in the morning. In stumbling out of bed and walking barefoot to the bathroom, you probably do more damage to the injured tendon than you might running the steeplechase. Often this simple intervention allows runners to cure their plantar fasciitis. In extreme cases, a podiatrist may need to prescribe a boot to immobilize the foot while in bed.

Achilles tendon injuries are similar to plantar fascia injuries in that they often are caused by overtraining, particularly speedwork if you wear spikes or racing flats with next to no heels. The Achilles tendon actually is the other and upper end of the heel, connecting it to the calf muscles above. Heel lifts can help. So can icing the injury several times a day and taking anti-inflammatories such as ibuprofen, a treatment that works for many if not most lower-body injuries. Achilles tendon and plantar fascia injuries hurt the most as you begin to run, then as your muscles warm, the pain sometimes will begin to subside, a sign that you can continue to run. If not, stop, limp back to your car, and make an appointment with a podiatrist to get properly diagnosed and treated.

A friend of mine from my early running days, Gordon Dickson of Hamilton, Ontario, suffered greatly from Achilles tendinitis. I finished second behind him in the 1958 Around the Bay Race, a 30-K in Hamilton 2 years older than the Boston Marathon. Gordy won that race five times. He offered me advice that I often pass on to others: "Never touch the tendon to see if it still hurts. It will, and all you are doing is irritating it, thus postponing your recovery." The no-touch advice worked for me the few times I suffered that injury, but not always for Gordy himself.

Ironically, I suffered a short bout of Achilles tendinitis while writing this book. Lori Nicholas, my massage therapist in Florida, one day pressed the left tendon too tightly, causing it to ache for several days. I don't blame her; the injury was about to happen anyway. Lori usually is good at preventing, ferreting out, and curing injuries rather than causing them. She applied equal pressure to the right tendon with no problems, but it seems that the left side of my body is, well, my "Achilles heel." The initial strain only lasted a few days, and I ran the 15-K Gate River Run soon after without pain, but a month later, I tripped over an uneven spot in the pavement while jogging with my daughter Laura in Detroit where we were gathered for a family wedding. Sometimes injuries can be caused by accidents as well as, or in addition to, overtraining. The tendon remained sore for nearly a week, but improved quickly so that I soon resumed running.

The worst Achilles tendon injury I witnessed occurred at the 1975 World Masters Championships in Toronto in 1975. Tom Sturak, a graduate of San Diego State whom I had first met at the 1952 NCAA Track and Field Championships, was running in the 800 meters. On the back straightaway, his Achilles tendon snapped, the sound so audible that we could hear it in the stands. It was like a shot from a gun. I've never told this story to another runner without having him cringe. After surgery, Tom was able to resume running, but not quite with the same élan.

AVOIDING INJURIES

If masters runners do suffer fewer injuries than our younger counterparts, it is because we have learned from our mistakes. When we make a training error and suffer an injury, we learn not to make that error again. But it may take years to accumulate the wisdom to injury-proof your body. If you are new to masters running, here are some tips to help you shortcut the learning process.

1. **Obtain proper equipment.** Few sports cost as little as running. Our main item of equipment is a pair of running shoes, costing less than $100 for most people. Fashionable clothing and fancy watches definitely are icing on the cake. Don't scrimp on footwear. Acquire shoes that are appropriate for your biomechanics. And when the shoes begin to show wear, throw them away. Most running injuries can be traced to the point where the shoe touches the ground.

2. **Train intelligently.** Don't just stumble from one workout to another, not knowing what you plan to run tomorrow, next week, next month, or even next year. Set goals, but give yourself time to meet those goals. If you don't have a coach, there are many training resources online, including schedules and answers to your questions.

3. **Find your red line.** Through trial and error, determine the point (usually miles run) at which you become overtrained or get injured. Then back your training down to a point below that red line. Sometimes you

Most running injuries are less threatening. It's not like football where a linebacker cracks back on you, and your knee is mush. Or like baseball, where you can get hit in the head with a fastball. Or like skiing, where a bad fall can cause knee damage requiring surgery. In fact, although I have no proof, I can trace at least some of my left-leg injuries to a bad fall on a black-diamond slope in Aspen, Colorado, when I was in college. Was it my left knee I injured? I suspect so. That injury caused me to reconsider whether someone whose main sport revolved around his legs should be participating in a sport such

can nudge this point upward by pushing on it gently, but everyone has a red line beyond which they get hurt. Find yours!

4. **Never get out of shape.** I offered those words of advice in an earlier chapter, but they bear repeating. Maintaining a solid base level of fitness means that when you want to increase your training to achieve a specific goal, you don't need to push too hard or too fast. Mileage increases should be made gradually.

5. **Keep a diary.** You don't need to record every workout in detail, but record trends, so that if you do get hurt you can look back and figure out why. Mileage trends are important, but so are activities around running. If you got hurt in a race, maybe it was because you jumped out of a car after a 4-hour drive just before competing.

6. **Utilize professionals.** If injured, and several days' rest doesn't result in a miracle cure, seek medical intervention. The runner's best friend is often a podiatrist, but other sports medicine experts from orthopedists to chiropractors to physical and massage therapists also offer healing hands.

Not all runners have bulletproof bodies. We all differ in our biomechanics and our susceptibility to injury. If you want to maximize your success and enjoyment as a runner, you need to give constant attention to avoiding injuries.

as downhill skiing. In fact, a number of runners who suffer injuries often can link cause-and-effect to previous injuries in other sports. Each year I warn those using my online programs to back off their participation in sports such as tennis, soccer, or volleyball, particularly as the long runs push into the double digits.

IDENTIFYING INJURIES

What are the injuries suffered most by masters runners? I asked that question in the online survey of that group done in cooperation with *National Masters News*. Here are the results, keeping in mind that respondents could check more than one injury, explaining why the numbers add up to more than 100 percent.

1. **Muscle pull—32 percent.** This would include any sudden pull, usually to a hamstring or calf muscle, that occurs during a race or workout. You might almost call this a sprinter's disease, since sprinters sometimes dramatically pull hamstring muscles in the middle of a 100- or 200-meter race, crumpling to the track in pain. Muscle pulls suffered by long-distance runners usually are less dramatic, though no less crippling. The day after running a 1500 heat at the 1999 World Masters Championships in Gateshead, England, I went hiking along Hadrian's Wall. Whether because of the race or the hike, my hamstring was so sore the next day, I had to scratch from my next race. There was no sudden pain, no crumpling onto the track. I just couldn't run full speed.

2. **Knee injury—30 percent.** Consider this the bad side of biomechanics. The knee is a very well designed joint unless you decide to run marathons. Do runners injure their knees more than nonrunners? Probably not. Orthopedists who do knee surgery admit that they operate more often on patients who are sedentary, whose problems stem from their being overweight, placing more strain on the knee joint. But anybody who has seen slow-motion photography of the stress transmitted to the knee with each stride cannot deny that this is an injury-prone

joint. Determining
the cause of knee
injuries often is fig-
uring out how and
how hard the foot
hits the ground.

> Most running injuries are minor. It's not like football where a linebacker cracks back on you, and your knee is mush.

3. **Plantar fasciitis—26 percent.** This might be called my injury of choice, given the fact that my favorite track event was
   the 3000-meter steeplechase. Pushing off the ball of the foot
   stretches the fascia running along the arch from the ball to the
   heel. Most often, pain is associated with the heel connection,
   but the connection at the ball can be strained, too. Hill running and speedwork most often cause this injury with recreational runners. Plantar fasciitis hurts the most right after you
   get out of bed in the morning, while your body is still stiff.
   Thus it's a form of morning sickness.

4. **Nonrunning injury—22 percent.** Not every injury suffered
   by masters runners is running-related. I've strained my
   shoulder or back lifting a suitcase or shoveling snow. Sitting
   long periods in a car causes me more hamstring problems
   than doing 100-meter repeats. Still, if you are overtraining,
   accompanying fatigue may make you more susceptible to that
   so-called nonrunning injury. If you hadn't run 50 miles last
   week, lifting a suitcase would not have been such a strain.

5. **Iliotibial band injury—20 percent.** This is the tendon that
   stretches across the side and front of the upper leg from the hip
   to the knee, and the pain can manifest itself either in the hip or
   knee connection. Unless you have been properly diagnosed by
   a sports medicine professional, you may not know that what
   you think is a knee injury is actually a strained iliotibial band.
   ("I don't care what you call it, Doc, just tell me how to fix it.")
   As with standard knee injuries, the cause is footstrike.

6. **Achilles tendinitis—17 percent.** For me at least, the causes
   of this injury often were the same as the causes for plantar

fasciitis, above. High mileage also can wear down the re-siliency of any muscle and stiffen ligaments and tendons. Lack of a careful warmup, particularly before speedwork, can also be a major cause. Because circulation is limited to this part of the body, it often takes a long time to cure this nagging injury. There are no instant cures.

7. **Shinsplints—16 percent.** I used to see this injury all the time when coaching high-school runners. If I limited my survey to those under 18, I suspect this injury would pop up to the top of the list. Orthopedists will tell you that "shinsplints" is a misnomer used to describe three or four injuries, but basically your lower leg aches so that running becomes uncomfortable, if not impossible. With high-school runners, the cause is a sudden increase in mileage among the youngest runners who don't run all summer, then go out for cross-country and try to keep up with those better trained. Beginning adult runners get shinsplints for the same reason.

8. **Stress fracture—9 percent.** Running being a lower-body ac-tivity, runners most frequently fracture their lower leg, although stress fractures sometimes can occur in the hip or foot. It's not like you have broken your leg, more like you have caused a small tear in the bone. It's a break you can feel, but not see. The tip-off as to whether you've suffered a stress fracture is if the pain is focused in one specific area about the size of a dime. Stress fractures don't appear immediately on x-rays and can be seen only several weeks later, when the healing process causes calcification of the bone. Too much mileage is the typical cause, although this could be said of many injuries.

9. **Health-related problems—8 percent.** Is catching a cold or coming down with the flu an injury? I would classify it as such, because you can't run as well with the former and prob-ably shouldn't run at all with the latter. Research suggests that marathoners more frequently catch colds the week before or

after their race, at a point when the high mileage depresses their immune systems. Various other illnesses also can be attributed to overtraining, for this same reason. Coming back from the Honolulu Marathon one year, I caught bronchitis, partly attributable to having run a hard 26 miles, but the person in the row behind me on the plane was coughing. It was an example of two causes coming together.

10. **No injuries—10 percent.** In some respects, I'm surprised that as many as 1 out of 10 respondents reported that they never got injured. Either they're in denial, or they haven't been running long enough or far enough. Sooner or later we almost all get hurt, particularly if our ambition causes us to do just a little bit more to achieve a PR. A few people, however, do have bulletproof bodies, and others have a higher tolerance for pain than others.

Those were the injuries reported in my survey of masters runners. John W. Pagliano, D.P.M., a podiatrist from Long Beach, California, shows a somewhat different and possibly more authoritative order of frequency based on a clinical study of more than 4,000 injured runners he has seen in his practice. Dr. Pagliano found that older runners had a disproportionately high number of foot and hip/lower back injuries than younger runners, who had a higher rate of lower leg and knee injuries. Less important than where your current injury rates on the hit parade is how you both prevent that and other injuries in the future and treat them if they occur.

Since Dr. Stan James identifies "training errors" as the most frequent cause of running injuries, the way to prevent them from happening is to not make errors. Easier said than done, you say, but maybe not. Smart training is the secret of injury prevention. Even by reading this book and taking note of the training advice within it, you already are one step ahead of the rest of the running population.

10 PROGRAMS

Do Masters Runners Need to Train Differently Than Others? Yes, We Do

s a younger runner, I sometimes trained frantically: running twice a day; covering more than 100 miles a week; a combination of long runs and short runs, fast runs and slow runs; workouts in the woods and on the track. This type of training was what it took to excel in the upper echelons of our sport. But the effort required to train that hard could be draining, both physically and psychologically. This was during an era, remember, when runners all were "amateurs" and prevented from accepting payment for our efforts. As much as possible, I tried to balance work and family obligations with my desire to become and remain a world-class runner, but I have to concede that sometimes it seemed that my life revolved around my running, rather than the other way around. And at times, running was not fun, or at least not as much fun as it should have been.

Decades past my peak accomplishments, I now view running from a different and perhaps more mature viewpoint. When motivated, I still can be intensively competitive, but I don't run two workouts a day any more. Sometimes I am lucky to run two workouts a week. One-hundred-mile weeks? That's a creature of the past. One hundred is more like my mileage for an entire month. When people ask me how many miles I now run, my typical answer lately has been "15 to

25 miles a week." And if you press me on the matter, I would probably concede 15 is closer to the truth than 25. My usual daily run is about 3 miles. That's the dis-

> You won't be able to perform the key, hard sessions well, and reap the most training benefits, unless you are well-rested before you do them.

tance I cover when I turn left at the end of my driveway in Long Beach and run a loop that takes me along the lakefront, past a golf course, and by homes with nicely manicured lawns shaded by tall trees. My favorite trail loop in Indiana Dunes State Park is about the same distance. Any more than that mileage I now consider a "long run."

The fact that I might run only two or three or four times a week now does not lessen my commitment to fitness. As described in the chapter on alternatives, I train in many different ways: everything from swimming to cycling to strength training. Walking has become a more important part of my agenda. Does the walk of nearly 2 miles I do each morning during the winter to purchase a newspaper count as training? Dr. Steven N. Blair of the Cooper Institute in Dallas probably would give me credit, but I don't record those miles in my diary.

If you strapped me in a chair, taped my eyelids open, and shined a bright light in my face, I probably would confess that after a hard run of 6 miles or more on pavement, my knees ache if I try to run the next day. (Please don't tell any nonrunners; they would simply say, "Suspicion confirmed!") But if I choose to swim or bike or walk on the beach with my wife on the second day, my knees feel fine on the third day. I enjoy the run more, particularly if I choose a soft surface like Ponte Vedra Beach or Indiana Dunes State Park.

Thus, I have modified my training programs to compensate for my age. All masters runners make at least minor modifications in their training as they move from their thirties into their forties, and modify it even more moving into their fifties and sixties. Once into our seventies and eighties, the modifications may need to be more severe. Would it bother me if forced to abandon running entirely and shift to walking? Again, don't tell the nonrunners, but I'm not sure it would. I'd still be outdoors and moving, enjoying the sights and sounds that, apart from any competitive goals, always have been the strongest motivational factor in my running.

In recent years, as I have moved from one decade of my life to the next, I have set celebratory goals to serve as a rite of passage. In 1991, I ran six marathons in 6 weeks to celebrate my 60th birthday. That task seemed too daunting 10 years later, so in 2001, I ran seven marathons in 7 months to celebrate my 70th birthday, also raising more than $700,000 for seven separate charities. I already have begun to look forward to my 80th birthday in 2011 and the possibility of running eight marathons in 8 years to celebrate that passage. That may or may not be achievable, so perhaps I should settle for running eight 8-K races in that length of time, particularly since one of my favorite races, the LaSalle Bank Shamrock Shuffle in Chicago, is that distance. As for my 90th birthday (if I reach that milestone), I haven't figured that one out yet.

Simply stated, modifications are necessary in any training programs if you plan to succeed. This is particularly true for masters runners. The standard programs don't always work for us. Either they are too easy, being designed for beginners, or they are too hard, being designed for young athletes who perhaps don't need as much recovery as we do between workouts. This is true, I confess, of the several marathon programs of mine that are available in books and online. Most popular and most successful is my 18-week Novice Marathon Training Program, which in addition to being available online also appears in my book, *Marathon: The Ultimate Training Guide*. Those who follow it rarely fail, but it is designed for beginners: people who have just begun to run or whose only goal is to finish comfortably. In ascending order of difficulty, I also offer four more marathon programs: Intermediate I, Intermediate II, Advanced I, and Advanced II. But those four programs feature 4 to 6 days of running, 40 to 55 miles a week. That may not be appropriate for masters runners.

With that in mind, I created a sixth program on my Web site for experienced runners who want to run only 3 days a week. It was designed primarily for: a) masters runners, b) heavier runners, or

SENIOR MARATHON TRAINING PROGRAM

Most training programs available in books and on my Web site feature 4 to 6 days of running a week. But not all runners can run that often. In his later years, George Sheehan, M.D., thrived on 3 days of running a week and even set a personal record of 3:01:18 in the 1979 Marine Corps Marathon at age 60. Many masters runners might be well-advised to follow Dr. Sheehan's example, since we do need more rest than younger runners after our hardest workouts, specifically the long runs while preparing for a marathon.

Keeping that in mind, I created the following Senior Marathon Training Program for older runners, also suitable for clydesdale (heavyweight) runners and those with tight time schedules. Warning: It is not a program for newcomers. At 12 weeks, it falls 6 weeks short of my usual 18-week marathon training programs. You need to already be fit to jump into a program that features in its first week a 12-mile-long run. But if you consider yourself a seasoned masters runner, it may work for you.

The three runs are scheduled for Tuesdays, Thursdays, and Sundays, the latter 2 days the longest runs. Mondays and Saturdays are rest days. I suggest strength training and stretching (S & S) on Wednesdays and Fridays, or you might want to cross-train on those days: swimming, biking, or walking. "Easy" refers to running at a pace comfortable enough to converse. "Pace" refers to running at your marathon race pace. There is nothing magic to this or any of my programs. Juggle the days to suit your convenience, remembering that the essence of this program is to run only 3 days—but make those running days meaningful.

c) runners with limited time to train. I called it my Senior Marathon Training Program, but it was by no means an easy program, nor was it for beginners. For one thing, the senior program lasted 12 weeks (not 18 weeks) and opened with a 12-miler on the weekend. And it ended with a 2-week (not 3-week) taper. That's not for novices!

And it may not work for all masters, many of whom still want to run more than three times a week and don't want to listen to

Week	Mon	Tue	Wed	Thu	Fri	Sat	Sun
1	Rest	4 mi pace	S & S	8 mi easy	S & S	Rest	12 mi easy
2	Rest	6 mi easy	S & S	6 mi easy	S & S	Rest	14 mi easy
3	Rest	4 mi pace	S & S	8 mi easy	S & S	Rest	12 mi easy
4	Rest	6 mi easy	S & S	6 mi easy	S & S	Rest	16 mi easy
5	Rest	4 mi pace	S & S	10 mi easy	S & S	Rest	12 mi easy
6	Rest	6 mi easy	S & S	6 mi easy	S & S	Rest	20 mi easy
7	Rest	4 mi pace	S & S	8 mi easy	S & S	Rest	12 mi easy
8	Rest	6 mi easy	Rest	Rest	Rest	Rest	Marathon

someone like me who suggests that they cross-train on other days of the week. A marathon training program certainly will not work if you want to limit your competitive goals to the 5-K, 10-K, or half-marathon. Lately, I have begun to look on that last distance as far enough for me, particularly since it now takes me as long to run 13.1 miles as it once took me to run 26.2 miles. The Senior Marathon Training Program does not work if you run track races more than road races. It will do little for you if you compete in field events. A few high jumpers and javelin throwers might have purchased copies of this book, since running is the base of all track-and-field events. Could I create specific training programs for each event on the track and field calendar? Yes, I could, but it would require another volume this size. Let me suggest instead a more radical approach:

You can create your own training program.

TRAINING PATTERNS

I'll show you how. Follow me as I describe the mental process I use while designing training programs for runners. I begin with a single week: 7 days, Monday through Sunday. What kind of training do I want you to do on each of those days? This creates a pattern that can be followed in expanding the program from 1 week to 4 weeks to 18 weeks or more. One marathon training program I developed with the help of Benji Durden of Boulder, Colorado, for my book *How to Train* lasts 84 weeks and encompasses two marathons plus 17 other races at shorter distances. That's an extreme example, but pick out any one week from Benji's program, and the pattern of workouts is the same, or very similar, to each of the other 83 weeks. There's a simple logic to the program that works very well—as long as you are a take-no-prisoners runner.

Start with the hard workouts. They are the key to any training program. First, ask yourself: How often do you want to run hard?

That's a vague term, since "hard" will vary from runner to runner. Hard can be determined either by distance or pace. A long run of any distance could be considered hard. Any workout where you run at, or near, race pace for any distance or length of time might be considered hard. For many runners, particularly those my age or beyond, simply getting out the door and running might qualify for designating a workout as hard.

For the January 1994 issue of *Runner's World,* I wrote a cover story on Bob Kennedy, an Indiana University graduate, who at that time was one of the top 5000-meter runners in the world. I attended the 1996 Olympics, where the most exciting track race was the 5000 in which Bob led up until the last lap, finally getting passed by a pack of Kenyans, failing to earn a medal but offering his best effort. A wave of noise rolled around the stadium with Kennedy

> All masters runners make at least minor modifications in their training as they move from their thirties into their forties, and modify it even more moving into their fifties and sixties.

and the leaders, following their every step for 12 and a half laps. I have attended Super Bowls and World Series and NBA and NCAA championship games and never have experienced a more riveting 13 minutes, the approximate length of time it took for that Olympic 5000.

Here's what I wrote in *Runner's World* about Kennedy's training: "In his normal training cycle, Kennedy schedules 3 hard days a week: Monday a stress day, Wednesday a semistress day, Friday a stress day. He trains on the track 2 of those stress days, once on the roads. Tuesday, Thursday, and Saturday are recovery days. Sunday, he runs long. In the racing cycle, the pattern is the same, except Friday is a rest day and Saturday a race."

Kennedy was coached then by Sam Bell, who also coached my son Kevin when he attended Indiana University a decade earlier. Kennedy told me: "The details [of my training] don't matter, as long as you do the work. The general philosophy of when to rest and when to go is most important."

That is what I mean when I use the word "pattern" in discussing how I, or other coaches, design training programs. Kennedy's training pattern is shown on page 202, ignoring the fact that, running twice daily, he also did each morning a "gentle tempo run" of 5 miles. "Gentle" to a world-class runner, of course, would not seem so to most masters runners. On days when he didn't run hard, Kennedy ran 7 miles in the afternoon. Here is a diagram of how he trained.

Week	Mon	Tue	Wed	Thu	Fri	Sat	Sun
1	Stress	Easy	Semistress	Easy	Stress	Easy	Long run

In the chapter on planning for peak performance in *Marathon: The Ultimate Training Guide,* I quoted Russell H. Pate, Ph.D., chairman of the Department of Exercise Science at the University of South Carolina (and also a 2:15 marathoner) as saying: "Figure out the key sessions you need for your program. Get them in there, then surround them with those kinds of recovery activities that allow you to continue over a period of time. Build your program on priorities. The highest priority is attached to the key, hard sessions."

For Bob Kennedy, those key, hard sessions would be Monday, Wednesday, and Friday, and some runners might consider Sunday's long run as a fourth hard day. This fits a pattern of 3 or 4 hard days a week. Compare this to the pattern of week 8 from my novice program for marathon runners.

Week	Mon	Tue	Wed	Thu	Fri	Sat	Sun
8	Rest	3-mi run	6-mi run	3-mi run	Rest	13-mi run	Cross-train

The numbers of miles are different. The days for hard runs (Wednesday and Saturday) are slightly different. The quality definitely is different on Kennedy's stress and semistress days and would be even for other fast runners following his program, but the pattern of hard and easy days remains the same.

CREATE YOUR OWN PROGRAM

Let's now begin to create a training pattern for a masters runner, using the same principles. Begin with 3 hard days.

Week	Mon	Tue	Wed	Thu	Fri	Sat	Sun
1	—	Run	—	Run	—	—	Run

We have not yet decided how many miles to run on those 3 hard days chosen for running, nor have we decided how fast to run those miles. This would vary too greatly from one master to another. Instead of deciding how many miles to run, consider how we might vary the pattern, purposely speaking in broad terms.

Week	Mon	Tue	Wed	Thu	Fri	Sat	Sun
1	—	Easy run	—	Fast run	—	—	Long run

Notice that with 3 hard days and 4 rest days—or at least 4 days that I have not yet defined—I have chosen to position 2 of those rest days between the two hardest of the three running workouts: the fast run and the long run. This allows you to both rest from the stress of the fast run and rest before the different but similar stress of the long run. Remember: You won't be able to perform the key, hard sessions well, and reap the most training benefits, unless you are well-rested before you do them. This is the theory of and rationale for hard/easy training.

Particularly as we grow older, it sometimes makes more sense to define our training in time rather than distance. The result might be called time-based training. Think minutes rather than miles. One advantage of time-based training is that you don't need to worry if you are running over a precisely measured course that allows you to measure how fast you are running. You can pick any road course or run in the woods at your pleasure. Of course, you could always purchase an electronic watch that uses satellite positioning to measure your exact distance run on any course, but we're old-timers not used to such fancy and expensive gadgets. Leave that GPS watch you got for Christmas home in its box. Here's how our working pattern would look with time-based training.

Week	Mon	Tue	Wed	Thu	Fri	Sat	Sun
1	—	45 min easy	—	30 min fast	—	—	90 min easy

Further defining what I mean by "30 min fast," the possibilities are infinite. For runners who followed my advanced

programs, I generally
suggest three types of
speed workouts: tempo
runs, interval training,
or hill repeats. Tempo

> Start with the hard workouts. They are the key to any training program.

runs typically are done on trails where the runner begins at an easy pace, then gradually accelerates to a hard pace, holds that pace for a few minutes, then gradually decelerates. Interval training usually involves fast repeats of anywhere from 200 to 1000 meters on a track, but could be longer repeats on the road. A hill repeat workout is similar to an interval workout on the track, except that instead of running hard and fast around an oval, then relaxing, you run hard and fast up a hill, then relax by returning downhill.

Even the fastest masters runners might not want to cram that much speedwork into a single week. Consider, however, this pattern for a 3-week period of time.

Week	Mon	Tue	Wed	Thu	Fri	Sat	Sun
1	—	45 min tempo	—	Hill repeats	—	—	60 min easy
2	—	45 min easy	—	Interval training	—	—	90 min easy
3	—	45 min tempo	—	45 min easy	—	—	120 min easy

That's a stiff dose of speedwork, appropriate only for the swiftest of masters runners. Let's consider a somewhat more gentle approach that removes so-called speedwork—although that doesn't mean you can't run somewhat faster than normal pace, particularly if we cut the time for one run a week, say on Wednesdays. And maybe it is time for me finally to define Mondays and Saturdays as days of rest.

Week	Mon	Tue	Wed	Thu	Fri	Sat	Sun
1	Rest	40 min easy	—	30 min fast	—	Rest	60 min easy
2	Rest	50 min easy	—	30 min fast	—	Rest	75 min easy
3	Rest	60 min easy	—	30 min fast	—	Rest	90 min easy

This leaves us with Wednesdays and Fridays on which I have as-signed no workouts. In my Senior Marathon Training Program on page 198, I reserved 2 days a week for strength training and stretching (S & S). Going to a fitness center and doing nothing more than lift weights is certainly one option. But many masters runners might enjoy adding different cross-training activities such as swimming or cycling, and I certainly feel that walking is an appropriate activity for masters runners. One good approach that I often follow is to cross-train for a half-hour and strength train and stretch for the other half-hour. If I train by biking or walking, I usually do my S & S workouts afterward, but if I choose swimming I do that afterward, since swimming can be very relaxing at the end of a hard workout in another sport.

Week	Mon	Tue	Wed	Thu	Fri	Sat	Sun
1	Rest	40 min easy	60 min bike	30 min fast	30 min swim	Rest	60 min easy
2	Rest	50 min easy	30 min swim	30 min fast	60 min walk	Rest	75 min easy
3	Rest	60 min easy	60 min bike	30 min fast	30 min swim	Rest	90 min easy

If that mix of running and cross-training doesn't appeal to you, create your own variation on the above training program. You are master of your own fate, or at least the training that leads to that fate.

THE END OF THE TUNNEL

Thus far, I have created patterns without any recognition that training most often is designed to prepare runners for a race, a so-called light at the end of the tunnel. Mindful of the training patterns I've suggested, consider now how you might modify these patterns to train for a 10-K race. Here is the Novice 10-K Training Program from my Web site, lasting 8 weeks. Remember, S & S on Mondays stands for strength training and stretching. Cross-training could be biking, swimming, cycling, walking, or any other aerobic activity.

NOVICE 10-K TRAINING PROGRAM

Week	Mon	Tue	Wed	Thu	Fri	Sat	Sun
1	S & S	2.5-mi run	30 min cross	2-mi run + strength	Rest	40 min cross	3-mi run
2	S & S	2.5-mi run	30 min cross	2-mi run + strength	Rest	40 min cross	3.5-mi run
3	S & S	2.5-mi run	35 min cross	2-mi run + strength	Rest	50 min cross	4-mi run
4	S & S	3-mi run	35 min cross	2-mi run + strength	Rest	50 min cross	4-mi run
5	S & S	3-mi run	40 min cross	2-mi run + strength	Rest	60 min cross	4.5-mi run
6	S & S	3-mi run	40 min cross	2-mi run + strength	Rest	Rest or 60 cross	5-mi run
7	S & S	3-mi run	45 min cross	2-mi run + strength	Rest	60 min cross	5.5-mi run
8	S & S	3-mi run	30 min cross	2-mi run	Rest	Rest	10-K race

That certainly follows the pattern of running on 3 days, cross-training on 2 or 3 days, and resting on 1 or 2 others, suggested as best for masters runners. An experienced masters runner, however, might want to cover more ground on the running days. I'm also going to use a time-based approach to this masters 10-K training program: prescribing minutes rather than miles. Another vari-

> You are master of your own fate, or at least the training that leads to that fate.

ation would be to save Monday for a day of rest and do the strength training and stretches on days already reserved for cross-training. Adding that extra day of rest may permit the addition of some speed-work. Since 71 percent of those answering my survey suggested they did speedwork, I know you want it. Is a single 10-K race in an 8-week period enough to keep most masters runners happy? Possibly not, so I added a midway 5-K race, should you choose to run it. Here's a 10-K program attuned to the needs of masters runners.

MASTERS 10-K TRAINING PROGRAM

Week	Mon	Tue	Wed	Thu	Fri	Sat	Sun
1	Rest	30-min run	30 min cross	Hill repeats	Rest	60 min cross	60-min run
2	Rest	30-min run	30 min cross	45-min tempo	Rest	60 min cross	65-min run
3	Rest	30 min run	35 min cross	Interval training	Rest	60 min cross	70-min run
4	Rest	30-min tempo	35 min cross	30-min run	Rest	Rest	5-K race
5	Rest	30-min run	40 min cross	Hill repeats	Rest	60 min cross	80-min run
6	Rest	30-min run	40 min cross	45-min tempo	Rest	60 min cross	85-min run
7	Rest	30-min run	45 min cross	Interval training	Rest	60 min cross	90-min run
8	Rest	30-min tempo	30 min cross	30-min run	Rest	Rest	10-K race

Don't like those numbers? Don't like that pattern? Don't want to think minutes; would rather think miles? By now, you should have a good idea of how I construct training programs for runners at all levels. Let's move on to the next level. Here's a training program to get you ready for a half-marathon race with a test 15-K en route. This assumes that you already have a strong fitness base or have just completed the 10-K program above.

HALF-MARATHON TRAINING PROGRAM

Week	Mon	Tue	Wed	Thu	Fri	Sat	Sun
1	Rest	45-min run	30 min cross	Hill repeats	Rest	60 min cross	60-min run
2	Rest	50-min run	30 min cross	45-min tempo	Rest	60 min cross	65-min run
3	Rest	55-min run	35 min cross	Interval training	Rest	60 min cross	70-min run
4	Rest	45-min tempo	35 min cross	30-min run	Rest	Rest	15-K race
5	Rest	55-min run	40 min cross	Hill repeats	Rest	60 min cross	80-min run
6	Rest	60-min run	40 min cross	45-min tempo	Rest	60 min cross	85-min run
7	Rest	60-min run	45 min cross	Interval training	Rest	60 min cross	90-min run
8	Rest	30-min tempo	30 min cross	30-min run	Rest	Rest	Half-marathon

What's the next step? Obviously it would be to move from the half-marathon up to the full marathon. My Senior Marathon Training Program on page 198 could help you to that goal. My Novice Marathon Training Program available online and in *Marathon: The Ultimate Training Guide* features 4 days of running a week, so it comes close to working for masters too, but here is a completely new Masters Marathon Training Program following the patterns established above. The key to any marathon-training program is the long run on the weekend, suggested here for Sundays. Get that right, and you should have no trouble in the marathon itself. The long run is prescribed in miles rather than minutes, since when it comes to running a 26-mile, 385-yard race, you do need to make sure you stretch your final training distance at least to 20 miles.

MASTERS MARATHON TRAINING PROGRAM

Week	Mon	Tue	Wed	Thu	Fri	Sat	Sun
1	Rest	30-min run	30 min cross	45-min run	Rest	60-min walk	6-mi run
2	Rest	30-min run	30 min cross	50-min run	Rest	60-min walk	7-mi run
3	Rest	30-min run	35 min cross	30 min run	Rest	60-min walk	5-mi run
4	Rest	30-min run	35 min cross	55-min run	Rest	60-min walk	9-mi run
5	Rest	30-min run	40 min cross	60-min run	Rest	60-min walk	10 mi run
6	Rest	30-min run	40 min cross	45-min run	Rest	60-min walk	7-mi run
7	Rest	30-min run	45 min cross	65-min run	Rest	60-min walk	12-mi run
8	Rest	30-min run	45 min cross	70-min run	Rest	60-min walk	13-mi run
9	Rest	30-min run	50 min cross	60-min run	Rest	60-min walk	10-mi run
10	Rest	30-min run	50 min cross	75-min run	Rest	60-min walk	15-mi run
11	Rest	40-min run	55 min cross	80-min run	Rest	60-min walk	16-mi run

(continued on page 210)

MASTERS MARATHON TRAINING PROGRAM (cont.)

Week	Mon	Tue	Wed	Thu	Fri	Sat	Sun
12	Rest	40-min run	55 min cross	60-min run	Rest	60-min walk	12-mi run
13	Rest	40-min run	60 min cross	85-min run	Rest	60-min walk	18-mi run
14	Rest	50-min run	60 min cross	60-min run	Rest	60-min walk	14-mi run
15	Rest	50-min run	60 min cross	90-min run	Rest	60-min walk	20-mi run
16	Rest	40-min run	50 min cross	60-min run	Rest	60-min walk	12-mi run
17	Rest	30-min run	40 min cross	45-min run	Rest	60-min walk	8-mi run
18	Rest	20-min run	30 min cross	2-mi run	Rest	Rest	Marathon

Similar to my other marathon-training programs, this one features step-back weeks with lesser long-run mileage to gather strength for the next push upward in distance.

Regardless of your race or distance, you can construct or modify your own training program following the patterns and principles suggested in this chapter. Even sprinters and field-event competitors can benefit from a training program that features 3 hard days a week for running. The necessary strength training can be done on the cross-training days. Most important in any training program is consistency. Never get too far out of shape. Blend speed, strength, and rest, and you will achieve success as a masters runner.

EPILOGUE

Masters runners dedicate their last decades to finding the perfect run

The epicenter for masters running, as age-group competition emerged in the mid-1960s, unquestionably was San Diego, California. David H. R. Pain lived in San Diego. He founded the first "masters mile" in San Diego. Pain organized the first track meet for athletes over 40 in San Diego. The first National AAU Masters Championships—the same meet in which I ran my first race as a master—was in San Diego.

The masters movement eventually spread to other parts of the U.S., to parts of Europe, and finally to most parts of the world, but San Diego was where it all began. It seemed that during the decade when the masters movement was germinating under the benevolent guidance of David H. R. Pain, I was constantly flying into San Diego as a reporter, a competitor, or both.

Strange how we recall vividly certain events while other events and activities—entire months, entire years—vanish almost as though they had not existed. One event that irrationally remains lodged in my memory is having viewed *The Endless Summer* at the Strand Theatre in Ocean Beach, the same suburb of San Diego where Pain had his law office. That town was and still is a hangout for surfers. The Strand, according to Ocean Beach resident Shel Dorf, had a very liberal policy not only about smoking, but also about what you smoked. "You could get high just sitting in the audience," says Dorf.

The Endless Summer, a 1966 documentary directed and narrated by Bruce Brown, was a half dozen years old when I first saw it, and I suspected it had been playing almost endlessly at the Strand for some time and would continue to do so as long as waves rolled onto the beach. The film followed two surfers as they embark on a journey to find "the perfect wave," starting in southern California and moving westward around the world, chasing sun, surf, and summer from Hawaii to Tahiti to New Zealand to Australia to South Africa, each stop offering both surfing ops and photo ops. Eventually, the pair discovered their perfect wave off a beach at Cape St. Francis, South Africa. Of course, the rationale for their trip and resulting film was not so much finding that wave, but rather the search for it.

"In surfing," says narrator Brown, "the object is to stay in the curl. All goes toward that." The "curl" is that rounded underside beneath the foaming lip of a wave in which the surfer hopes to maintain position, knowing that a miscalculation, a shift in balance, will send him and his board tumbling toward oblivion. On only one occasion did I sample surfing, renting a board during a vacation to the Outer Banks in North Carolina, where the waves, admittedly, loomed much less frighteningly than those at Cape St. Francis. After being slammed into the sand several times, I decided that running served as a more satisfactory activity for someone of my abilities.

But in many respects, *The Endless Summer* existed as an allegory for my life as a masters runner—and maybe yours: our journey to find the perfect run in what we hoped would be an Endless Autumn.

It is true that as runners and as individuals, we move through different seasons: from spring to summer, from autumn to winter. In the spring of our lives, we are children engaged in what Dr. George Sheehan referred to as "play," running from one game to another. We run because it is fun, not to beat people, not to win prizes or age-group trophies, and certainly not because of a desire for "physical fitness," an abstract concept youngsters cannot comprehend.

As we become adults in the greening summers of our lives, we abandon play and focus on completing our educations, breaking free from our parents, obtaining good jobs, enjoying the pleasures money can bring. We get married. We become parents ourselves. We settle into relationships and routines that signal the end of summer. But as we move into the autumns of our lives, at least some of us revert to childish pursuits and embrace exercise as a means of bringing quality to our lives as well as to extend those lives.

We seek to delay as long as possible the winter of our discontent. In at least its allegorical sense, winter is not fun. It is cold. It is dark. It is a prelude to the grave. If we cannot avoid winter, we would like at least to postpone it, to shorten it, to redirect its harshest winds, to negate winter's effect on our ability to enjoy life to its fullest.

In becoming masters runners, we seek an endless autumn. And like surfers chasing the sun westward around the world, we hope our journey never will end while knowing that someday it will. As long as we find ourselves capable of taking one running step, we exist in an endless autumn.

As I completed work on this, my 34th book, in the 73rd autumn of my life, I traveled once more to San Diego. I called David H. R. Pain. We agreed to meet with our wives at a restaurant in Ocean Beach, not far from his former law office, not far from the movie theatre where I first viewed *The Endless Summer.* Sadly, the Strand Theatre is now gone, replaced by a souvenir shop.

The night was filled with pleasant conversation. David seemed recovered from a bicycle accident that temporarily had blunted his relentless pursuit of fitness. I described running a few months earlier in the National Masters Championships in Decatur, Illinois, finishing far behind. I wondered whether I could muster the motivation to improve my time and position at the next World Masters Championships in Spain. If not, two years later I would move into a different age group with its new set of opportunities and challenges. Can I reignite the competitive fires that led me to four world titles and numerous national titles and records?

Maybe, and maybe not.

While seasons repeat themselves, allegorical man is allowed only one cycle: one movement through spring to summer, from autumn to winter. There is no endless summer, or endless autumn, except in the eyes of documentary filmmakers and poets.

Reflecting on my own career as a runner, spring ceased that moment when I sat on the infield grass at the 1952 NCAA track meet and learned from wiser runners that there were better ways to train. So began a summer of triumphs and failures, performances good and bad, as I competed at the highest levels of my sport. Then came the masters years, the autumn of my competitive life, extended as I moved from age group to age group to age group, where you grow inexorably slower, but it matters not. To move is to live. Now is not yet the time to enter a winter of discontent. Light the fires once more! I have many trails yet to tread, many races yet to run.

Good luck to all of you who embrace the masters life, who seek an endless autumn.

ACKNOWLEDGMENTS

Jeremy Katz, executive editor of Rodale Books, first suggested to my agent, Angela Miller, that I write a book on masters running. Although over the years I have done several books that touched on the subject of aging (specifically *Fitness after Forty,* 1976, and *Masters Running Guide,* 1990), none had either the scope or the focus of the book you now hold in your hand.

After agreeing to the project and while contract negotiations continued, I visited Rodale's offices in Emmaus, Pennsylvania, and met with Jeremy and editor Heidi Rodale. We decided that the book should be directed at runners over the age of 40, both motivating them and telling them how to train. Other than that, I was free to write. Originally, I thought I might write this book in the third person, almost as a guide. But because I had been involved, almost from day one, as both competitor and reporter in the masters movement started by David H. R. Pain, I found that the first person worked best. And as I showed the manuscript to Jeremy and Heidi, they agreed with this approach. I thank them for their collaboration on *Masters Running.* Thanks also to Angela Miller, who was responsible for bringing the three of us together. Angela has worked with me on most of my recent running books, both initiating ideas and checking the fine print in contracts.

At Rodale, kudos also to project editor Kathy Dvorsky, who supervised the journey from manuscript to bound book. And to Drew Frantzen, who designed the text and cover.

All during the writing, I stayed in close contact with Suzy Hess and Jerry Wojcik at *National Masters News.* Thank you also to Al Sheahen, that publication's founder, and to Peter Mundle, keeper of masters records. Dozens of others provided facts when needed; their names are sprinkled throughout this book. Amby Burfoot at *Runner's World* offered encouragement through frequent e-mails.

Without the support of my wife, Rose, and our family, I never could have continued my career as a masters runner. (Our son Kevin now competes in masters track meets.) Finally, if David Pain in 1966 had not come up with the idea of a "masters mile" for runners over 40, a book with the title *Masters Running* never could have been written, nor would running be as much fun as it is now.

INDEX

Underscored page references indicate boxed text.

ABOUT THE AUTHOR

Few other writers have combined their professions and passions as successfully as Hal Higdon. *Masters Running* is Higdon's 34th book. Many of these books are on running; others are on subjects as diverse as the Civil War, business, and true crime. One children's book was made into an animated film for TV. In addition to being *Runner's World*'s most prolific contributor since its founding in 1966, Higdon also has written for *Reader's Digest, National Geographic, Playboy,* and the *New York Times Magazine.* In 2003, the American Society of Journalists and Authors gave Higdon its highest honor, the Career Achievement Award.

While forging a career in journalism and raising, with his wife, Rose, a family of three children (they now have nine grandchildren), Higdon continued to run, placing fifth in the 1960 Olympic trials and fifth (first American) in the 1964 Boston Marathon.

But Higdon's greatest successes came as a masters runner, beginning with a victory in the 10,000 meters at the National AAU Masters Championships, 3 days after his 40th birthday. He went on to win four world masters championships. His times winning M40 and M45 world titles in the 3000-meter steeplechase remain American records as of this printing, 3 decades later. His 5000 time remained an American masters record for nearly a quarter century.

Higdon lately has shifted much of his writing to the Internet, providing InterActive training programs for the 5-K to the marathon on his popular Web site, www.halhigdon.com.